# The
# Every Other Day
# Diet

# Introduction

*Welcome to the Every-Other-Day Diet*

## CUT BACK TODAY – CUT LOOSE TOMORROW!

*D*iets *don't work.*

You've probably read that statement dozens of times, if not hundreds. But even though 'Diets don't work' has become a truism, it's not true. The truth is *diets don't work when you diet every day*. Diets don't work because no one can endure day after day of deprivation, cut off from the foods they love. Diets don't work because no one can follow their complex and artificial rules for weeks and months on end. Diets don't work because they're unworkable!

But the reasons why traditional diets *don't* work are the

same reasons why the Every-Other-Day Diet *does* work – because it does away with daily deprivation and hard-to-follow rules. And you don't have to just take my word for it, because unlike other diets, the Every-Other-Day Diet has years of rigorous scientific research to back up its claims.

Having done a PhD in nutritional science and as an associate professor of nutrition at the University of Illinois, I've spent the last ten years conducting weight-loss studies on *modified alternate-day fasting* – a simple and science-proven approach to quick, permanent weight loss and lifelong weight maintenance. I've distilled that decade of systematic, successful research into a practical plan, which I'm presenting for the first time in this book, *The Every-Other-Day Diet*.

I want to take a moment to also introduce my co-author, Bill Gottlieb, CHC, the author of 12 other health books that have sold more than two million copies worldwide, a health coach certified by the American Association of Drugless Practitioners and the former editor in chief of Prevention Magazine Books and Rodale Books.

Bill not only brought his writing skills to *The Every-Other-Day Diet*; he also brought his skills as a veteran health journalist, working with me to find the latest scientific research, reported throughout the book. This book is infused with Bill's passion and professionalism as a health coach dedicated to the wellness of his clients and his readers.

In this introduction, I'll explain the difference between the Every-Other-Day Diet (the EOD Diet, for short) and the other diets out there. I'd also like to tell you my own story of losing weight by dieting every other day. Then I'll provide a brief overview of the contents of the book and how to use it for weight-loss success.

So let's get started with a closer look at the crucial differences between every-day dieting and the Every-Other-Day Diet.

## FORGET ABOUT DIET DEPRIVATION – WELCOME TO DIET SATISFACTION

Every-day diets are typically about deprivation – what you *can't* eat. They tell you what *not* to do, handing down the dieter's equivalent of the Ten Commandments, like

- Thou shalt not eat more than 10 per cent fat.
- Thou shalt not eat more than 1½ oz (40g) of carbohydrates.
- Thou shalt not eat meat.
- That shalt not eat wheat.
- Thou shalt not eat sugar.
- Thou shalt not covet thy neighbour's sugar.

So you try to obey your diet's unique set of commands, whether there are ten or 100 of them. But you end up feeling frustrated. So you 'sin'. You eat 'bad' foods. You feel like a 'bad' person. And then you repent. ('I'll never eat doughnuts again!') And then, inevitably, you repeat the whole self-defeating cycle all over again.

Why does this happen? As day follows night, dietary excess always follows dietary deprivation. When a food is forbidden, it becomes tantalisingly tempting, and you crave it. Are you on a low-carb diet? You're probably craving pizza. On a low-fat, plant-based diet? You're probably dying for a steak. On a Paleo Diet? You're probably dreaming about cheese enchiladas. Eventually, you give in to those cravings. Maybe you even binge.

Another reason diets fail: hunger. Hunger is good. Hunger is *natural*. Hunger is your body's way of telling you that it needs fuel. The point of hunger is to let you know it's time to take in more calories. But weight-loss diets are about calorie restriction. (In spite of all the claims to the contrary by diet gurus who favour high or low quantities of carbs, protein and/or fat, it's *always* calorie restriction that powers a diet's ability to help you shed pounds.) So when you diet, you feel hungry. Maybe even cranky. Maybe even depressed. Nobody can deal with daily hunger and its accompanying emotional stress for long. The Every-Other-Day Diet solves this problem by making sure that you don't feel chronically deprived.

Diets also present you with a complex and daunting set of rules to be obeyed – or else. They tell you *what* you can and can't eat. They tell you *how much* you can and can't eat. They often tell you *when* you can and can't eat. All those rules end up ruling your life. And that's no fun. So what if you could drop pounds and still . . .

## Eat all you want!

The Every-Other-Day Diet makes losing weight easy. There's no long-term deprivation and there's one simple rule:

**Eat 500 calories on the day you diet (Diet Day), and eat anything you want and as much as you want the next day (Feast Day).**

No keeping track of carbs, fat or protein. No avoiding any particular food; all foods are allowed. No complex meal plans. And, yes, you diet only *every other day*. As I discuss at length in chapter 1, my research shows you lose just as much weight on the EOD Diet as when you're on an every-day diet.

With every-other-day dieting, dietary deprivation never lasts longer than a day, and total dietary freedom is always just a day away. Now, you may be thinking to yourself, 'There's no way that's going to work. I'm going to eat so much on Feast Day that I'll never lose weight.' But the studies I've conducted show that overeating on Feast Day *doesn't* happen. On average, people following the Every-Other-Day Diet eat about 110 per cent of their normal caloric needs on Feast Day. And they eat about 25 per cent of their normal caloric intake on Diet Day. That's an average of nearly one-third fewer calories over two days – and a perfect formula for steady, safe weight loss.

Why don't EOD dieters binge on Feast Day? Because they're not feeling deprived! When you're on the Every-Other-Day Diet, you know you'll be able to eat whatever food you want, and all the food you want, every other day. You don't have to eat 'like there's no tomorrow' because there's a tomorrow right around the corner, and another one soon after that. The Every-Other-Day Diet solves the problem of diet *deprivation* through diet *satisfaction*.

## MY PERSONAL STORY OF WEIGHT-LOSS SUCCESS ON THE EVERY-OTHER-DAY DIET

In this book you'll read many first-hand stories from participants in my studies on the Every-Other-Day Diet, people who were officially classified as 'obese' (about 2 stone 2lb (13.6kg) or more overweight) and who typically lost 1 stone 6lb (9.1kg) or more. But before I introduce you to those people, I'd like to tell you my own story.

I've never had that much weight to lose, but, like most people, I sometimes struggle with extra weight. In the past, I tried to lose that weight with every-day calorie restriction. But the diet that I find works best for me is the same diet I've been studying for nearly a decade, the Every-Other-Day Diet. Here's what happened . . .

Back in 1996, at the age of 17, I was on my school swimming team, working out for two hours at a time, up to ten times every week. I needed a lot of calories to fuel those workouts (and my growing body), and I ate a lot. But I never had a weight problem. I was 5'7" (1.7m), 9 stone 9lb (61.2kg), muscular and strong. When I got to university, I stopped swimming competitively, but I kept on eating the same amount of food as I had in school. It never occurred to me that the number of calories needed to power my workouts would be too many for my somewhat sedentary scholastic lifestyle. And so I gained about 1 stone 1lb (6.8kg) – the classic freshers' weight gain.

Fortunately, I was studying in nutrition, so I was learning for the first time about calories and healthier food choices. With that new knowledge, I started eating more sensibly, and slowly but surely I lost the weight I'd gained. By late in my sophomore year, I once again weighed 9 stone 6lb (61kg). And that's right where my weight stayed until I was 31 years old and got pregnant.

The final trimester of my pregnancy coincided with the festive season. I found myself at party after party, feeling free to eat anything and everything I wanted to eat. (No one judges you for your appetite when you're pregnant!) As a result, I ended up gaining a little more weight than my obstetrician would have preferred, putting on about 2 stone 12lb (18.1kg), rather than the suggested 1 stone 11lb–2 stone 7lb (11.3–15.9kg).

After my baby was born, I expected to easily lose that extra weight. And why not? Shedding extra pounds had been a breeze back at university. But I was in for an unpleasant surprise. Just over half of those extra pounds did come off quickly, which is pretty typical after a pregnancy. But the rest? They stuck around. And I felt stuck.

Finally, after a couple of months, I put myself on a 1300-calorie-a-day diet. And after six difficult months of daily deprivation, my weight was back down to normal. At that point, I figured the weight would stay off without my having to think about it. Wrong again. Over the next six months or so, the weight crept back on until I was at 10 stone 4lb (65.3kg). I couldn't believe it! I was eating healthily. I was walking regularly. But here I was, overweight again.

Believe me, I didn't want to go back on a 1300-calorie-a-day diet for months and months, endure the daily struggle and hardly see the scales budge week after week. I was ready for a different approach. And so I started using the very same weight-loss method I'd been studying – the alternate-day modified fasting of the Every-Other-Day Diet. And like the participants in my studies, I loved it. I didn't have to diet every day. I could eat whatever I wanted to every other day and I could eat as much as I wanted to. Best yet, I saw *immediate* results, quickly losing the weight I wanted to lose. I'm back to my original weight. And if I see the scales start to creep up by a couple of pounds – well, I just go on the Every-Other-Day Diet for a week or two and the weight comes right off.

The Every-Other-Day Diet has worked for me. It has worked for hundreds of participants in my studies, all of whom have been officially obese. And I'm sure it will work for you, a certainty I think you'll share after you read chapter 1 of this book, which presents the scientific evidence showing the effectiveness of the Every-Other-Day Diet. I feel quite passionate about my work and research, given the stakes: obesity is one of the biggest and most harmful health plagues of our time.

## It's Time for a Revolutionary Approach

The week I was finishing writing *The Every-Other-Day Diet*, the American Medical Association (AMA) decided to officially recognise obesity as a *disease*. (As a medical term, 'obesity' is a reflection of body mass index, or BMI, a measurement of body fat. Medically, you're 'overweight' with a BMI of 25 to 29.9, and 'obese' with a BMI of 30 or over, which is generally 2 stone 2lb (13.6kg) or more overweight.) I certainly understand why the AMA made that decision.

Just about all of the participants in my scientific studies have been obese and I know how difficult life can be for them. There's the discomfort of all those extra pounds. There's the struggle with self-esteem. And then there's the poor health: research links obesity with many other health problems, including heart disease, stroke, type-2 diabetes, cancer, osteoarthritis, gout, liver disease, sleep apnoea and depression.

In the UK just under a quarter of men (24 per cent) and just over a quarter of women (26 per cent) are obese (with another 41 per cent of men and 33 per cent of women being overweight), A quarter of all adults in Australia are obese (with a further 35 per cent being overweight). The statistics are similar in New Zealand where 28 per cent of adults are obese (with a further 37 per cent being overweight). World-wide, 1 in 6 adults is obese. That's hundreds of millions of people worldwide who are weighed down by extra pounds – and my sincere hope is that going on the Every-Other-Day Diet helps them.

I began conducting research on modified alternate-day fasting because I knew that overweight and obesity were taking such a significant toll on the lives of so many people, and I saw that conventional, every-day diets were failing to help them.

I was looking for a new way, a better way, to help people lose weight, and then to help them keep it off for a lifetime. My scientific research on both weight loss and weight maintenance shows that the every-other-day approach to weight control offers just the help overweight and obese people need. And I am delighted that now you'll be able to make practical use of my research by reading about and following the Every-Other-Day Diet and shedding those excess pounds for once and for all.

## How to Use This Book

Like the Every-Other-Day Diet itself, this book is simple to use. I suggest you do the following:

***Start by reading chapter 1***, which tells you about the scientific findings that support the EOD Diet. Chapter 1 will fill you with confidence and enthusiasm about this unique weight-loss programme.

***Next, read chapters 2 and 3*** to familiarise yourself with Diet Day (500 calories) and Feast Day (unlimited calories). Once you've read them, you're ready to start the EOD Diet. But before you do, it will help to . . .

***Check out chapter 4*** for Diet Day ideas. This chapter offers 28 400-calorie lunches, 28 400-calorie dinners and 28 100-calorie snacks – all quick and easy to prepare, and all delicious.

***Read chapter 5 to turbocharge the EOD Diet with exercise.*** This chapter looks at my research on combining EOD dieting and exercise to help you lose more weight and lose it faster.

***Keep the weight off with chapter 6.*** In this chapter, you'll find the Every-Other-Day Success Programme, a scientifically proven way to keep off the weight you've lost. That's crucial, because five out of six dieters regain all their weight after one year. I'm happy to say that weight regain is unlikely to be your fate if you follow the EOD Success Programme.

## WELCOME TO FAST, EASY AND PERMANENT WEIGHT LOSS

The Every-Other-Day Diet is simple and straightforward.

The Every-Other-Day Diet is easy.

The Every-Other-Day Diet is scientifically proven to *work*.

You'll lose weight fast and reach your goal weight.

You'll keep the weight off.

And you'll do so while eating all the food you want and any food you want, every other day.

Ready to get started? Just turn the page.

## CHAPTER 1

# The New Science of Every-Other-Day Dieting

*Study after study shows the
Every-Other-Day Diet really works*

When it comes to health and wellbeing, there's a reason we look to the accuracy and authority of scientific experiments to help us work out what's truly useful and sound information as opposed to the baseless, specious and fad claims and advice that's out there – to separate the proverbial wheat from the chaff: *scientific experiments aren't based on hype and hope.*

A well-designed, well-conducted scientific experiment helps separate truth from wishful thinking, fact from fantasy. And a *series* of scientific experiments, testing the same theory and generating the same results (what scientists call *replicating* a scientific finding), creates a body of knowledge you can *trust* and then *act on*.

Given the importance of weight loss to our health and wellbeing, to preventing and reversing disease and to restoring self-esteem, you'd think most diet books would be packed with scientific evidence that justifies their approach. But that's *not* the way it is.

Yes, there have been scientific studies on a few popular diet plans. For example, a study published in the *Journal of the American Medical Association* showed that overweight and obese women on the Zone Diet, the low-carb Atkins Diet or the low-fat Ornish Diet lost a little bit of weight after one year of dieting – an average of 3½lb (1.6kg) on the Zone Diet, 4.8lb (2.2kg) on the Ornish diet, and 10.4lb (4.7kg) on Atkins.[1] (Yes, that's after dieting for *one year.* I think you'll do a lot better on the Every-Other-Day Diet.) However, most popular weight-loss plans don't have any scientific support for their approach. None. Zero. Zilch.

Why am I making such a big fuss over scientific support for the diet plans in diet books? Because the Every-Other-Day Diet *does* have a significant body of scientific research behind it. To date, I've conducted seven clinical trials involving nearly 400 people, and I have published the results in 20 scientific papers. My studies have shown, again and again, that the Every-Other-Day Diet *works.* The people in my studies lose weight. And in my ongoing, three-year study on weight maintenance sponsored by the National Institutes of Health, EOD dieters are keeping the weight off.

In other words, the Every-Other-Day Diet is a research-proven diet that you can *trust.* If you follow this diet, eating

500 calories on Diet Day and whatever you want on Feast Day, the scientific evidence says you *will* lose weight. And if you go on the maintenance programme described in chapter 6, the Every-Other-Day Success Programme, my newest findings show you *will* keep the weight off.

I know the Every-Other-Day Diet may seem too good to be true. I know you might be asking yourself, 'Can I really lose weight eating anything I want, every other day?' Never fear. You can. And not just because I say so – because nearly a decade of rigorous scientific research says so. And since your trust in the science-proven effectiveness of the Every-Other-Day Diet is so important to me, I've devoted this chapter to sharing the research and studies that support my claims. I want you to know – really *know* – that the diet you're about to undertake isn't a novel idea that's never been put to the test. It's not based only on the experience of patients in one doctor's practice (which is the case with many diet plans). And it's not theoretical – an idea that seems to make metabolic and biological sense, but has little real-world evidence to show that it works.

By learning about the science of every-other-day dieting and by reading about my studies and their positive findings, you can embark on this new weight-loss programme with confidence, conviction and enthusiasm. So let's start at the beginning: with my discovery of this diet, in the basement of a building at the University of California, Berkeley, where, in 2006, I was a postdoctoral fellow.

## THE MICE THAT ALWAYS LOST WEIGHT

After I graduated from McGill University in Canada with a PhD in nutrition, I moved to California to do postdoctorate research in the Department of Nutritional Science at Berkeley. (A native Canadian, I was delighted to discover that 'winter' in Northern California is just a series of rainstorms and that daffodils bloom in February!)

Under the guidance of my advisor, Dr Marc Hellerstein, I investigated the effects of calorie restriction on cancer. There was already a lot of research on calorie restriction and longevity in animals; it showed that when mice are fed less food, they live up to twice as long as mice fed a normal diet. Furthermore, some of the biochemical mechanisms triggered by calorie restriction in longevity research are known to be anti-cancer. The mechanisms include slower cell division; lower levels of IGF-1 (insulin-like growth factor 1, a growth factor that stimulates cancer cells to divide and multiply); and lower levels of glucose, the main fuel for cancer cells.

Our research question was this: can you put a mouse on the ultimate form of calorie restriction – fasting – so that the growth of cancer cells is slowed, but the animal does *not* lose weight? (In their research, scientists are always trying to isolate and analyse specific factors. In this case, we wanted to isolate the effect of *calorie restriction* on cancer from the effect of *weight loss* on cancer.)

But as hard as we tried, we couldn't keep the mice from losing weight! We fasted them one day and let them eat all they wanted the next day. But they never ate enough calories on 'feed day' to compensate fully for the total lack of calories on 'fast day'. Sometimes they managed to eat 150 per cent of a normal day's calories on feed day. Sometimes they ate up to 170 per cent. But they never ate 200 per cent of their normal caloric intake on feed day to make up for the zero calories on fast day. And so they *always* lost weight.

My experiment had failed because there was no way to separate the effect of calorie restriction from the effect of weight loss. I was not a happy scientist! But a scientific investigation that seems like a dead end can suddenly present a new vista of opportunity. And that's just what happened: I had a eureka moment, an *Aha!*, a conceptual breakthrough when I realised that the mice always lost weight on alternate-day fasting. The mice *always* lost weight. Could alternate-day fasting help us *humans* lose weight? If people fasted one day and then ate all they wanted the next day, would they always lose weight, just like the mice?

The concept of the Every-Other-Day Diet – using alternate-day fasting for *weight loss* – was born. It was time for me to say goodbye to the mice in the basement at Berkeley and move to Chicago, where I had been hired as an assistant professor in the Department of Kinesiology and Nutrition at the University of Illinois at Chicago. There, I started conducting studies on weight loss. With people.

## THE MAGIC NUMBER

When I looked closely at the scientific literature on alternate-day fasting for cancer and heart disease – studies conducted exclusively on animals in the laboratory – I found that many of the risk factors for the two diseases were lowered most effectively when the animals ate only 25 per cent of their normal calories on fast day. Not 75 per cent. Not 50 per cent. Not 0 per cent, or a total fast. Time and again, the healthiest percentage was 25 per cent or what I call a *modified fast*.

And the 25 per cent level of calories on fast day did more than prevent and reverse signs of disease. It also prevented the loss of muscle mass the animals otherwise had experienced at 0 per cent, when they were given no food on fast day.

Why was that important? Losing muscle mass while dieting is a disaster for weight loss and weight maintenance. That's because muscle (*lean body mass*, in scientific terms) is metabolically active tissue that burns a lot of calories. Lose muscle during dieting and you'll burn fewer calories after dieting and regain your weight – as fat! This is perhaps the key reason why 5 out of 6 people who lose weight gain it all back (and then some). So I decided that on fast day – the day called *Diet Day* in the Every-Other-Day Diet – people would eat 25 per cent of their normal caloric intake, or about 500 calories. I was ready to recruit participants and begin my study.

At this point, I have to make an embarrassing confession: even though I was about to conduct a study on every-other-day dieting in people, I didn't think the diet would work!

Why not? Well, many overweight people eat around 3000 calories a day, and I couldn't imagine they'd be willing or able to eat only 500 calories every other day. And then there was my conversation at a medical conference with Dr Eric Ravussin, PhD, director of the Nutrition and Obesity Research Center at the Pennington Biomedical Research Center at Louisiana State University. I told him I was thinking of conducting a study on alternate-day fasting for weight loss, allowing my participants to eat 500 calories on fast day.

'Don't even bother,' he said. And then he proceeded to tell me (to my surprise) that he and his colleagues had recently conducted a human study on alternate-day fasting, in which the participants ate zero calories on fast day. A study that didn't go too well.[2] First, he wasn't able to recruit anyone from outside Pennington to participate in the study, because the idea of fasting every other day seemed so onerous; he was forced to enrol Pennington professors in the study. Next, he couldn't even convince many of those professors to participate for all three weeks of the study. Of the 16 that started, only 8 finished. And even those who finished told him they hated alternate-day fasting. Their families hated it, too. 'I was so cranky and irritable on fast day that my wife wouldn't talk to me,' said Dr Ravussin, who participated in his own study.

I had already planned to allow my study participants to eat 500 calories on fast day; my conversation with Dr Ravussin convinced me I'd made the right decision. For successful every-other-day dieting, you need to be on a *modified fast*, not a total fast. (In scientific papers, I sometimes call my approach ADMF, or alternate-day modified fasting.) You need to eat a small meal during the day, so you can stay balanced emotionally and mentally, interact with people without blowing a fuse, and get through your working day efficiently and effectively.

In spite of my doubts, I went ahead with my study, recruiting people who were normal weight and overweight (not obese). My goals for the study were broad: to find out if anyone could actually stay on the diet for a few months, and if they would lose weight. Much to my surprise, they did both!

There were 32 people in the original study.[3] Sixteen went on the Every-Other-Day Diet. The other 16 were the *control group* – they didn't diet or change their eating habits at all. After three months, my colleagues and I compared the two groups. Not surprisingly, people in the control group didn't lose any weight. But all of the every-other-day dieters shed pounds.

Participants who were normal weight at the start of the diet lost an average of 11.9lb (5.4kg) after three months. Those who were overweight lost an average of 11lb (5kg). (A few of them lost as much as 1 stone 11lb (11.3kg).) The overweight group also saw significant drops in bad cholesterol (low-density lipoprotein, or LDL) and in high blood pressure. And most of the participants said they didn't find the diet difficult at all.

I had proven to myself that every-other-day dieting was a reasonable, effective approach to weight loss. People *could* eat 500 calories every other day on Diet Days, without difficulty. People *could* eat whatever they wanted on Feast Day and still lose weight.

As you can imagine, I was very excited about this first set of results. After all, just about everybody hates daily dieting. Don't you? You hate the endless weeks and months of non-stop deprivation. You hate the constant hunger. You hate the complicated requirements and rules. That's why you've probably given up most of the diets you've started. Who wouldn't? Daily dieting is a drag. But every-other-day dieting is a new and effective way for people to lose weight – *without* deprivation, *without* hunger, *without* rigid rules.

After the success of this first study, there were many other questions about every-other-day dieting that I wanted to answer, with detailed, careful and repeated research:

- Would the diet work on the obese, or would they binge on Feast Day?
- How hungry would obese people be on the diet? So hungry they couldn't help but overeat?
- Could people exercise on Diet Day? And would they overeat when they exercised?
- Would the diet work if you ate high-fat food? Or was low-fat food the only way to go?
- How would the diet affect risk factors for heart disease like total cholesterol, LDL cholesterol, HDL cholesterol and high blood pressure?
- How would the diet affect hormones like leptin, which play such a key role in appetite?
- Was there a way for people who lost weight on the Every-Other-Day Diet to *maintain* their weight loss?

Nearly a decade later, after six more studies on people and more than 20 published scientific papers on every-other-day dieting, I'm proud and delighted to say that these questions have been answered. In fact, it's only *because* they were answered that I feel comfortable presenting the Every-Other-Day Diet to the tens of millions of people who *really* want to lose weight and keep it off and not just be disappointed by another every-day diet.

Let's take a closer look at a few of my studies and what I discovered. To make it easier for you to follow the trail of my research, I've listed the year each study was published, the journal it was published in and the specific findings of the study.

## BODY MASS INDEX – THE WAY SCIENTISTS MEASURE OVERWEIGHT

As you read the studies in the rest of the chapter, you'll encounter several common, every-day terms: *normal weight* . . . *overweight* . . . and *obesity*. However, nutritional scientists and other health experts use these terms in a very specific way: to indicate the level of *body mass index*, or BMI, a standard measurement of body fat. The three main categories of BMI are

*Normal weight: 18.5 to 24.9*
*Overweight: 25 to 25.9*
*Obese: 30 and above*

How do these three levels of BMI translate into actual pounds? Here are two examples: A 5'4" (1.63m) woman a healthy weight up to 10 stone 5lb (65.8kg), overweight between 10 stone 6lb (66.2kg) and 12 stone 6lb (78.9kg) and obese above 12 stone 6lb (78.9kg). A 5'10" (1.78m) man is a healthy weight up to 12 stone 6lb (78.9kg), overweight between 12 stone 7lb (79.4kg) and 14 stone 12lb (94.8kg) and obese above 14 stone 13lb (94.8kg).

To work out your BMI, use the BMI calculator at the NHS Choices website:

http://www.nhs.uk/tools/pages/healthyweightcalculator.
aspx

Just enter your height in feet and inches or in metres, and
your weight, and then hit the 'Calculate' button. I'm happy
to say my BMI is 21.6; Bill's is 22.4. The Every-Other-Day
Diet for weight loss and the Every-Other-Day Success Programme for weight maintenance (which you'll read about in
chapter 6) helps both of us stay in the normal range.

## 2009, *American Journal of Clinical Nutrition*
*The Every-Other-Day Diet works and is super-healthy, too!*

A study in the *American Journal of Clinical Nutrition* was the
first to definitively show that every-other-day dieting works to
help obese people lose weight.[4]

My colleagues and I studied 16 obese people, 12 women
and 4 men, with an average weight of 15 stone 3lb (96.8kg)
and an average BMI of 33.8. All of them went on the diet for
two months. For the first month, they ate frozen and other
packaged foods for their 400- to 500-calorie lunches and
100-calorie snacks on Diet Day. (We distributed the lunches
and snacks on a weekly basis.) For the second month, they
prepared the Diet Day lunches and snacks themselves, after
meeting with a nutritionist on our staff who counselled them
about the calorie level of Diet Day and the foods and portion
sizes that would help them stay at that level. (You'll find all
the practical details for Diet Day in chapter 2.)

The results:

***An average of 12lb (5.4kg) of weight loss.*** After two months, the average weight loss was 12.3lb (5.6kg), a steady, healthy weight loss of 1.5lb (0.7kg) per week. And the rate of weight loss was just about the same whether the participants were given frozen and packaged food or they prepared their own food. They just kept losing pounds, week after week.

***Dieters lost fat, not muscle.*** Our EOD dieters also lost most of their weight as *fat* – 11.9lb (5.4kg), on average, meaning that they shed only a few ounces of muscle. Losing fat rather than muscle is crucial in successful weight loss, because muscle burns calories. A typical dieter on other plans sheds 75 per cent of her weight as fat and 25 per cent as muscle; the typical EOD dieter sheds nearly all of her weight as fat. That's probably one reason why my subsequent studies have shown that EOD dieters, unlike most other dieters, don't regain the weight they lose.

***Their BMI fell.*** The average BMI also dropped to 29.9. Many people who were classified as *obese* at the start of the study were now classified as *overweight*. That's a significant and health-giving improvement: as BMI decreases from obese to overweight, so does a person's risk for many diseases, including heart disease (obesity doubles risk), diabetes, arthritis and cancer.

***There was very little cheating.*** Our records showed that, on average, the dieters managed to meet the 500-calorie requirement of Diet Day for about 9 out of 10 Diet Days throughout the two months of the study. This showed me that the Every-Other-Day Diet is a diet people *could* and *would* follow at home.

***Cholesterol plummeted.*** We also saw big decreases in

total cholesterol (21 points) and LDL cholesterol (25 points), lowering the risk for heart attack and stroke.

***Dieters had lower blood pressure.*** Systolic blood pressure (the upper number of the blood pressure reading, reflecting arterial pressure when the heart pumps blood) dropped, on average from 124 to 116. Lower blood pressure means a lower risk for heart attack or stroke.

***Dieters had a slower heart rate and a stronger heart.*** The participants also saw a startling drop in average heart rate, from 78 beats per minute to 74 – a sure sign of a stronger, healthier heart.

***My scientific conclusion:*** the Every-Other-Day Diet is an 'effective diet strategy to help obese individuals lose weight and to confer protection against coronary artery disease'. That's what I wrote (in the formal, restrained language of scientific discourse) in the *American Journal of Clinical Nutrition*.

For this book, I'll also state my conclusions about my studies a little more personally and enthusiastically: the Every-Other-Day Diet works – and it's really good for you, too!

---

## PAUL'S STORY:
## 'I'VE GOT TO CHANGE MY LIFE'

*Weight loss: 2 stone 13lb (18.6kg)*

The evidence was conclusive for Paul Hussein, an international lawyer living in London and Switzerland. At 6 feet (1.8m) tall and 15 stone 4lb (97kg), he was guilty of being overweight, and that extra fat - from eating a lot, and eating mostly high-fat food - was destroying Paul's health. His heartburn was so bad he had to take an antacid with every meal. He suffered

*(continued)*

from back pain. He had sleep apnoea and snored. He felt tired all the time. He had type-2 diabetes and was on a medication to control his blood sugar. And he was a bowel cancer survivor.

In August 2012, Paul was watching the BBC documentary *Eat, Fast and Live Longer*, which featured my research on alternate-day modified fasting (the scientific term for every-other-day dieting) along with other methods of intermittent fasting. He told us what happened next.

'I said to myself, "That's enough. I need to change my life – for myself, and for my wife and children. I need to go on a diet and lose weight."'

Paul decided to go on the two-day-per-week pattern of dieting used by Michael Mosley, the programme's host: a 500-calorie modified fast on any two days of the week, with unrestricted eating the other five days.

But the diet didn't work.

'I couldn't get a grip on my eating by fasting just two days a week,' Paul told us. 'I overate so much on the days I wasn't fasting that I didn't lose *any* weight.'

So Paul went on the Every-Other-Day Diet. And this time, modified fasting worked. After nearly a year on the diet, Paul weighs 12 stone 5lb (78.5kg) – a loss of 2 stone 13lb (18.6kg)!

'One day of fasting followed by one day of feasting is the perfect diet for me,' he said. And weight loss isn't the only positive change that Paul has experienced. His heartburn went away. He stopped snoring. His back pain is better. His blood-sugar level has normalised and he no longer needs to take diabetes medication. And at his most recent check-up for bowel cancer, the doctor gave him a clean bill of health.

'I also find that I'm thinking a lot more clearly when I'm in court,' he said. 'And I don't feel tired during the day like I used to.'

We asked Paul what he liked to eat on Diet Day. 'I eat a simple vegetable soup, or perhaps a small piece of chicken with a serving of whole grain like quinoa and I feel very good after that meal. If I feel hungry on Diet Day, I drink a glass of water, or distract myself with another activity.'

'Every-other-day dieting has now become my daily life and I don't think I will ever give it up.'

## 2010, *Nutrition Journal*

*Bingeing doesn't happen, hunger stops and physical activity isn't a problem.*[5]

Now I knew that every-other-day dieting *worked* for obese people. But I wanted to know more details about the diet:

- How hungry did people get on Diet Day, and was hunger a problem for trying to stick with the diet?
- Were people bingeing on Feast Day?
- Were people so physically depleted on Diet Day that they engaged in less physical activity?

To learn the answers to these questions, I analysed some of the data from my first study more closely. I discovered the following:

**There was no overeating on Feast Day.** I thought the

obese participants in my study would eat a lot more on Feast Day to make up for the caloric restriction of Diet Day, but they didn't. On average, the dieters ate the same number of calories they always ate (and even a little less), consuming an average of 95 per cent of their normal caloric intake on Feast Day. In other words, Diet Day was *not* followed by Overdo-It Day!

***Hunger vanished.*** My colleagues and I asked the study participants to rate their hunger on the evening of each Diet Day, using a scale of 0 to 100; 0 was 'not at all' hungry, and 100 was 'extremely' hungry. After three weeks of dieting, the average ranking was 60. After four weeks, it was 50. And after seven weeks it was 35. In fact, after about two weeks on the Every-Other-Day Diet, most of the participants said they felt little or even no hunger on Diet Day. That's more good news, because it's constant, gnawing hunger that drives most people to cheat on or give up a diet.

***Satisfaction with the diet increased week by week.*** Meanwhile, over the eight weeks of the study, satisfaction with the Every-Other-Day Diet went up and up. Using the same 0 to 100 scale, the study participants reported a satisfaction level of 35 in the first weeks of the diet, but a satisfaction level of 50 by week eight. In other words, their good feelings about being on the diet – and no doubt their pride in the results as pounds kept peeling off – increased week by week. I'm pretty sure you'll have the same experience.

***Physical activity wasn't a problem, even on Diet Day.*** We measured the level of physical activity throughout the study by asking the participants to wear a pedometer, a device that measures the number of steps taken every day.

Two thousand steps is about one mile, and most of us take between 4000 and 7000 steps a day.

I thought the study participants would feel less energetic on Diet Day and would take fewer steps. But that wasn't the case. The average number of steps on Diet Day and Feast Day were almost the same: 6416 on Diet Day, and 6569 on Feast Day. This was more good news: the Every-Other-Day Diet doesn't slow you down!

***My scientific conclusions:*** 'These preliminary data offer promise for the implementation of alternate-day fasting as a long-term weight-loss strategy in obese populations,' I wrote in *Nutrition Journal*. I had made many additional discoveries about the Every-Other-Day Diet:

- Obese people could limit their food intake to one low-calorie meal and one snack per day and not overeat the next day.
- Hunger disappeared after two weeks or so on the diet.
- Physical activity didn't decrease on Diet Day.
- Weight loss was steady, constant and significant.

My next and very important question: could this diet help prevent and reverse heart disease? The answer, as you'll read in a moment, was an unqualified *yes*.

## 2010, Obesity

*The Every-Other-Day Diet helps prevent and reverse cardiovascular disease – one of the UK's biggest killers.*

In my first study, the participants not only lost weight; they gained health.[6] Specifically, they gained added protection against heart disease:

*A 21 per cent decrease in total cholesterol.* Their total cholesterol dropped from 175 to 138mg/dL, for an average decrease of 21 per cent. Every 1 per cent drop in total cholesterol lowers the risk of heart disease by 2 per cent, which means the Every-Other-Day Diet lowered the risk of heart disease by a whopping 42 per cent. Not a bad 'side effect' of successful dieting!

*A 20-point drop in LDL cholesterol.* LDL is the type of cholesterol that can build up on an artery wall and clog the artery, causing a heart attack or stroke. After eight weeks, the study participants had an average drop in LDL from 102mg/dL to 72mg/dL. This took them right to the 70mg/dL level that doctors try to achieve in patients at risk for heart disease by prescribing a cholesterol-lowering statins. (Personally, I'd rather lose weight than take a statin, since these commonly prescribed drugs are linked to fatigue, muscle pain, memory loss and other health problems.)

*Triglycerides fell from 125mg/dL to 88mg/dL.* Like cholesterol, triglycerides are a blood fat that can raise your risk of heart disease. The study participants went from the 'normal' to the 'optimal' level of triglycerides, as defined by the US government's National Cholesterol Education Program.

*Systolic blood pressure fell from 124 to 116mm Hg.* Eight points might not seem like much of a decrease, but it meant the difference between some of the study participants being prehypertensive – just below the level where a person would be diagnosed with outright high blood pressure – and having a normal blood pressure level, below 120.

**My scientific conclusion:** 'Alternate-day modified fasting may decrease the risk of coronary heart disease in obese individuals,' I wrote in *Obesity*, the world's leading scientific journal on the topic, in 2010. Given that heart disease causes over 70,000 deaths every year in the UK, that's a very important finding.

---

## THE EVERY-OTHER-DAY DIET IS SAFE

Over the years, I've often been asked about the *safety* of the Every-Other-Day Diet – after all, 500 doesn't seem like very many calories. Is it so few calories that EOD dieters could harm themselves in some way?

After studying hundreds of people on the EOD Diet, I'm happy to say that I've never seen a *single* health problem caused by the very low caloric intake of Diet Day or by the unlimited eating of Feast Day. Not one.

In fact, I've seen just the opposite. Risk factors for heart disease normalise. Total and LDL cholesterol go down. Triglycerides decrease. Blood pressure is lower. Most importantly, of course, the pounds peel off – anywhere from 1 to 5lb (0.5-2.3kg) per week, depending on how heavy the dieter was when he started the diet. And extra pounds are linked to a higher risk for dozens of different conditions and diseases, including cancer.

At the same time, unlike people on most other diets, the dieter doesn't lose calorie-burning muscle – and that retained muscle not only powers faster weight loss during

*(continued)*

the diet, but also sets the stage for post-diet weight maintenance. Many studies have linked increased lean body mass (muscle) to better health – even to longer life. So rather than posing a threat to health, the Every-Other-Day Diet improves it dramatically.

Of course, if you've got a chronic health condition like diagnosed heart disease, type-2 diabetes or cancer, or if you're on any prescription medications, particularly drugs for controlling blood sugar, *you must check with your GP or specialist before starting the Every-Other-Day Diet or any weight-loss programme.*

The EOD Diet (like most weight-loss diets) is not intended for pregnant women or women trying to get pregnant. It's also not for anyone with type-1 diabetes, where a modified fast might be harmful.

What about kids and teenagers? More than 30 per cent of young people in the United States are now either overweight or obese. Could they benefit from the EOD Diet? The modified fast of the Every-Other-Day Diet isn't appropriate for the growing bodies of kids. However, I'm hoping to develop and study a version of the Every-Other-Day Diet for teenagers. Stay tuned, Mum and Dad!

**Bottom line:** the Every-Other-Day Diet is safe for just about all adults.

## 2012, Metabolism[7]

*The Every-Other-Day Diet works even when you eat high-fat foods!*

In my first two studies on every-other-day dieting, participants ate low-fat foods on Diet Day – because low-fat foods like fruits, vegetables, whole grains and beans provide more filling bulk for fewer calories. But most people *don't* eat a low-fat diet. Just the opposite. They eat a high-fat diet, with 35 per cent to 45 per cent of calories from fat.

Since I wanted the Every-Other-Day Diet to work for everyone, I needed to find out if it could work for people who eat a high-fat diet on Diet Day while still maintaining the 500-calorie limit. To that end, I conducted a study with 32 obese people, putting them on the Every-Other-Day Diet for eight weeks. On Diet Day, 16 people ate high-fat foods that delivered 45 per cent of calories from fat. The other 16 ate low-fat foods, with 25 per cent of calories from fat. We prepared the foods for both groups, to guarantee their fat content.

The results:

***Those eating high-fat foods on Diet Day lost MORE weight than those eating a low-fat diet!*** That's right: after eight weeks on the diet, those eating high-fat foods had lost *more* weight than those eating low-fat food: 9.5lb (4.3kg), compared to 8.2lb (3.7kg).

***They had trimmer tummies.*** Both low- and high-fat groups trimmed nearly 3in (7.6cm) off their waistlines. Dietary fat didn't make anybody fatter.

***They had healthier hearts.*** Both groups had healthy decreases in total cholesterol, LDL cholesterol and triglycerides.

***My scientific conclusion:*** 'An alternate-day fasting/high-fat diet is equally effective as an alternate-day fasting/low-fat diet in helping obese subjects lose weight and improve coronary heart disease risk factors,' I wrote in the journal *Metabolism*.

Why did the people eating a high-fat diet lose more weight? Well, they were slightly less likely to go off the diet on Diet Day, cheating 13 per cent of the time, compared to 22 per cent for the low-fat dieters. And I think it's likely they stuck to the diet *because* it was high-fat and therefore more enjoyable and satisfying.

**Bottom line:** the Every-Other-Day Diet works even if you eat high-fat foods on Diet Day. When it comes to weight loss, it's not fat that makes the difference. Or carbohydrates. Or protein. It's *calories*. Stick to the 500-calorie limit on Diet Day and you *will* lose weight.

## 2013, Obesity[8]

*The combo of EOD dieting and exercise is unbeatable for weight loss and a healthy heart.*

My first studies found that people didn't become less physically active when they were on the Every-Other-Day Diet, on either Diet Day or Feast Day. A modified fast didn't modify their capacity to move around. But, I wondered, what would be the effect of combining the Every-Other-Day Diet and *exercise* – not just daily physical activity, but a regular workout? Would people lose more weight than they would by dieting alone? Would their hearts be even healthier? My next study on the Every-Other-Day Diet attempted to answer those questions, by comparing people who went on the EOD Diet to people who went on the EOD Diet *and* exercised.

You can read all about this study in chapter 5, 'Every-Other-Day Dieting and Exercise', but here's the super-positive bottom line: at the end of the study, those people who went on the EOD Diet and exercised had twice as much weight loss, had more muscle, banished more tummy fat, lowered LDL cholesterol and raised HDL cholesterol. The diet-alone group had only lowered LDL cholesterol.

***My scientific conclusion:*** the combination of the Every-Other-Day Diet *and* exercise 'produces superior changes in body weight, body composition [muscle and fat] and lipid [blood fat] indicators of heart disease risk, when compared to individual treatments,' I wrote in *Obesity*.

Or, to put it less scientifically and more plainly: if you want the best results, go on the Every-Other-Day Diet *and* exercise.

## 2013 'ObesityWeek' (a presentation at the yearly scientific conference of the Obesity Society, which publishes the journal *Obesity*)

*My NIH-sponsored research shows that the Every-Other-Day Success Programme works – with this post-diet programme, you don't regain the weight you just lost!*

As I've pointed out several times in this chapter, the sad fact of weight loss is that it's rarely permanent. In a study published in the *International Journal of Obesity*, only 3 per cent of people studied maintained their weight loss after five years. Other studies are a little more positive (but not much); they estimate that 80 per cent to 90 per cent of dieters regain all their weight.[9]

Unfortunately, most diet books ignore this fact. Or they make an enthusiastic but baseless pronouncement about how you'll maintain your weight after the diet. They might as well be telling you to believe in Santa Claus. I think any diet book that doesn't give you a scientifically-proven, evidence-based programme to *maintain* yourself at the weight you reached on the diet – and that's just about every diet book out there, including most of the other diet books on intermittent fasting – is setting you up for disappointment, not to mention the health problems that can go with regaining the weight you've lost. *The Every-Other-Day Diet* isn't that kind of diet book. It includes the Every-Other-Day Success Programme, which you'll read about at length in chapter 6.

In November 2013, several months after completing the writing of this book, and six weeks before its publication, I reported the preliminary results of that study at the annual 'ObesityWeek' conference, the world's most prestigious conference on obesity and weight loss.

***Dieters had only 1lb (0.5kg) of regained weight.*** In the first six months of the study, people were on the Every-Other-Day Diet, and many lost a lot of weight (up to 3 stone 3lb (20.4kg)). In the next six months, those who were on the EOD Diet went on the EOD Success Programme. My preliminary results showed that they regained an average of *1lb (0.5kg)*. Meanwhile, the control group – people who went on a standard, every-day, calorie-restricted diet for six months and then went off it – regained an average of 5lb (2.3kg).

I'm also happy to say that all the heart-healthy benefits of the Every-Other-Day Diet – lower LDL cholesterol, lower triglycerides, and less tummy fat – were maintained during the EOD Success Programme. The participants also had lower levels of blood sugar and insulin, a sign that they were less prone to developing type-2 diabetes.

It's been a long journey from that basement at Berkeley to a three-year, multimillion-dollar study sponsored by the National Institutes of Health; from the lightbulb moment of having a fresh idea to the light at the end of the tunnel for millions of people who have failed to lose weight on other diets, or who have shed pounds only to see their weight return.

My comprehensive research shows that the Every-Other-Day Diet is a wholly unique and effective way to lose weight and keep it off without daily deprivation, without hunger and without complex and hard-to-follow rules. My research also shows the diet can help prevent and reverse several risk factors for cardiovascular disease, one of the biggest causes of death in the UK. And with all this positive research under my belt, I am very comfortable making you a promise about the weight you will lose on the EOD Diet.

## WEEKLY, MONTHLY AND TOTAL WEIGHT LOSS: THE EOD PROMISE

I'm sure you have one big question at this point: just how much weight can I lose on the Every-Other-Day Diet? Well, I am happy to report that you can lose:

*12lb (5.4kg) per month.* In my most recent research, many EOD dieters lost up to 12lb (5.4kg) in the first four weeks of dieting, or 3lb (1.4kg) per week – the promise on the cover of this book.

*Up to 3 stone 8lb (22.7kg).* In my two- and six-month studies, some EOD dieters lost up to 3 stone 8lb (22.7kg).

Of course, there's no *guarantee* you'll lose weight on the EOD Diet. In my studies, the rate of weight loss depended on how heavy my participants were when they started (the heavier you are, the more you lose); their level of motivation; and even the time of year when the study was conducted (it's harder to lose over the festive season). But if you eat 500 calories on Diet Day and whatever you want on Feast Day and stick to that pattern, it's nearly a certainty that you *will* lose weight at a steady rate, until you reach your weight-loss goal, whether that's losing 10, 25, 50, or 100 pounds or more.

And when you have reached your goal, it's time to implement the Every-Other-Day Success Programme, the lifetime approach to keeping off the weight you just lost. You'll find the practical details of the Success Programme in chapter 6. So what are you waiting for? Let's get started!

---

### EOD – EASY AS 1-2-3!

1. The Every-Other-Day Diet has years of rigorous *scientific testing* behind it.
2. The Every-Other-Day Diet is *evidence-based*.
3. The results of the Every-Other-Day Diet are *real*.

## CHAPTER 2

# Diet Day

## 500 calories is easy, when it's every other day

Like other nutritional scientists, when I write up my studies for publication in journals, I almost never use the word *calorie*. Instead, I say *energy*, because that's what a calorie is: the amount of energy required to raise the temperature of one kilogram of water by one degree Celsius. Yes, a calorie is a measurable unit of heat, of energy, of *fuel*. If you ingest more calories than your body can burn, you store them (usually as fat) – and you gain weight. If you ingest fewer calories than your body needs to function, your body burns calories – and you lose weight.

Calories are the merciless mathematics of a food, of a meal – of a slim life or a lifetime struggle with weight. And so we *count* calories, using books and apps and food labels and menus. And we *miscalculate* calories, gobbling up a low-fat food to shed pounds while overlooking the fact that it's sometimes loaded with high-calorie sweeteners. And we *debate* calories; a handful of experts claim that calories in some macronutrients like carbs burn differently from calories in others like protein or fat, spawning endless variations of low-carb/high-protein or high-carb/low-protein diets.

I think all those diets are high fad/low results. As a scientist who has devoted her professional life to studying calorie restriction, I can tell you with 100 per cent certainty that if you eat food that contains less energy (calories) than your body requires, you will burn stored energy (calories) and lose weight. That's a scientific fact, like the law of gravity. Call it the Law of Calorie.

The Every-Other-Day Diet helps you obey the Law of Calorie in a completely new way. The Every-Other-Day Diet doesn't ask you to know and track the exact amount of calories in every food and beverage you ingest. (Good luck with that.) The Every-Other-Day Diet doesn't ask you to deprive yourself of calories every day, leaving you feeling hungry and frustrated. The Every-Other-Day Diet has one simple-to-follow, calorie-based rule:

> **Eat 500 calories one day (Diet Day) – and eat whatever level of calories you want the next day (Feast Day).**

This chapter presents the practical details of Diet Day: how to go successfully through the day with minimal (or no) hunger and maximum ease. Want to start burning calories and losing weight? There's no time like Diet Day.

## How Low Can You Go?

When you're not on a diet – when your every-day pattern of eating is aimed at *maintaining* weight – you probably consume somewhere between 2000 and 2500 calories a day. In the UK the Scientific Advisory Committee on Nutrition (SACN) estimated average requirements for calories for adults over 18 years old are 2,079 calories for women, and 2,605 for men. For older adults who are no longer mobile energy requirements may be lower, and alternative energy intake values for lower levels of activity have also been estimated.

When you go on a diet – when you want to burn more calories than you consume and shed pounds – you submit to the eating pattern nutritional scientists call *calorie restriction*, usually limiting your daily intake to 1000 to 1500 calories a day. Some dieters, however, decide to consume even *fewer* calories. Why?

Maybe they're extremely obese, with over 7 stone (44.5kg) to lose. Maybe they want to lose weight very quickly. And so they go on a *very low-calorie diet* (VLCD), with a daily intake of about 800 calories.

And then there's the Every-Other-Day Diet, where, on Diet Day, you consume 500 calories. Is that doable? Is that even *safe*? Yes and yes. Surprisingly, 500 calories can provide a lot of hearty eating: one (or even two) satisfying meals a day, along with a snack. Find that statement hard to believe? Just check out the tasty recipe and meal suggestions in chapter 4. You'll soon find that Diet Day is very doable and very delicious.

Some people feel hungry on Diet Day for the first week or

two of EOD dieting. (Later in this chapter you'll find plenty of tips to help you get through the hunger pangs of those first few weeks.) But my studies show that the hunger quickly resolves: the people in my studies report they *don't* feel hungry on Diet Day after two weeks or so on the diet. Hunger just goes away.

***Bottom line:*** the experiences of hundreds of EOD dieters show that one day of modified fasting isn't all that hard – particularly when it's followed by a day of all-out dietary delight.

## WHY 500 CALORIES?

As I discussed in chapter 1, my first scientific studies on alternate-day fasting for weight loss – the genesis of the Every-Other-Day Diet – were on mice. These studies tested many different levels of alternate-day calorie restriction, trying to determine the perfect level for healthy weight loss. I tried 75 per cent of normal caloric intake; 50 per cent; even 0 per cent – a total fast. And the winner was 25 per cent.

At 25 per cent, the mice had the *maximal* amount of weight loss with the *minimal* level of muscle loss. In other words, they lost fat but not muscle. And retaining muscle while dieting is a must for health and long-term weight maintenance. Also, 25 per cent of calories also produced the best improvements in risk factors for heart disease and type-2 diabetes.

Subsequently, my studies on people have confirmed that 25 per cent is the perfect percentage for every-other-day dieting: 500 calories, if you normally eat 2000 calories a day. At that percentage, you lose weight quickly, steadily and healthily.

Obviously, 25 per cent of normal caloric intake is a different number for different people. If you're a 6'3" (1.9m) man weighing 14 stone 9lb (93kg), the normal level of calories you burn is a lot different from a 5'2" (1.6m) woman weighing 10 stone 10lb (68kg) pounds; the bigger the person, the more calories needed to maintain weight. In my scientific studies with groups of people, we carefully determine 25 per cent of normal caloric intake for each study participant, using a precise formula and double-checking it with a sophisticated medical test.

Unfortunately, I can't offer you that kind of individualised determination of 25 per cent of your normal caloric intake; it's just not possible outside of a highly controlled scientific experiment. But here's the good news: an individualised version of the EOD Diet is *not* required for it to work. Why not? Because my studies have allowed me to determine a consistent average caloric intake on Diet Day: 480 calories for women and 520 calories for men. You don't need a degree in mathematics to figure out the average of those two numbers is 500. Which means that

- 500 calories on Diet Day is the average intake among the hundreds of people who have participated in my studies and successfully lost weight;
- 500 calories is the *scientifically-proven* level of calories for efficient weight loss; and
- 500 calories is the level that *works*, no matter what you weigh when you start the Every-Other-Day Diet. And you should weigh yourself when you start the diet and every day thereafter.

## EIGHT TIPS TO MAKE DIET DAY WORK FOR YOU

### Tip 1:  Weigh Yourself Every Day

How often should you check your weight when you're on the Every-Other-Day Diet? In my studies, we encouraged the participants to weigh themselves *every day*, and to average the weight of the most recent Diet Day and Feast Day. For example, if you weigh yourself the morning of Diet Day and you weigh 10 stone 8lb (67.1kg) and you weigh yourself the morning of Feast Day and you weigh 10 stone 10lb (68kg) your current weight is 10 stone 9lb (67.6kg).

Why do I think you should weigh yourself every day? Maybe you've heard that you *shouldn't* get on the scales every morning, because it can be discouraging to discover you haven't lost much weight, or that it keeps your focus on short-term success rather than on permanent weight loss. But that's not what scientific studies show. They are *pro*-scales. Here are some very revealing results:

***After one month of weighing, participants had 3lb (1.4kg) extra of weight loss.***[1] When researchers at the Minneapolis Heart Institute studied 100 obese people over six months, they found that people lost *1lb (0.5kg) more* for every 11 days they self-weighed. In other words, if you weigh yourself every day for a month, you lose about 3lb (1.4kg) more than people who don't. In fact, those who self-weighed were *ten times more likely* to lose at least 5 per cent of their body weight during the six months of the study. 'Self-weighing may be a strategy to enhance ... weight-loss programs,' wrote the researchers in the *American Journal of Preventive Medicine*. I agree!

When those same researchers reviewed 12 studies on self-weighing and weight loss, they found that 11 of the studies showed that self-weighing was linked to more weight loss and better weight maintenance, and also to not becoming overweight in the first place.

***Daily weighing doubles weight loss.*** In a two-year study of more than 1200 obese people conducted by scientists at the Marshfield Clinic Research Foundation in Wisconsin and reported in the *International Journal of Behavioral Medicine*, those who weighed themselves daily lost more than twice as much weight as those who weighed themselves monthly.[2]

***People average 347 fewer calories per day when they weigh themselves that day.*** A team of scientists from the University of North Carolina studied 91 overweight people for six months, in an experiment focused on self-weighing.[3] Those who weighed themselves daily ate an average of 347 fewer calories per day than those who weighed themselves weekly. They also lost a lot more weight – 1 stone 3lb (7.7kg) compared to four-fifths of a pound! The researchers also noted that the study participants who weighed themselves just about every day *liked* doing so. I think you will, too, as your scales give you the most important and positive feedback of all: you are steadily losing the weight you want to lose! But weighing yourself daily is important not only for *losing* weight. It's also important for *maintaining* weight loss.

***If people didn't weigh themselves regularly, 4.5 times more weight was regained.*** Researchers in the Department of Psychology at Drexel University conducted a one-year study on 3000 people who had lost 2 stone 2lb (13.6kg) and kept it off for one year and reported their findings in *Obe-sity* in 2007.[4] At the start of the study, 36 per cent said they weighed themselves at least once a day, and those who did so had the lowest body mass index (BMI, a standard mea-surement of body fat – see p. 22). They also scored highest on psychological tests measuring the ability to make rational choices about eating.

A year later, the researchers found that the change in the rate of self-weighing after the start of the study – whether or not the participants weighed themselves with lesser or greater frequency during the year of the study – was an *exact match* for the amount of weight regained:

- Those who self-weighed *less* regained 9lb (4.1kg).
- Those who self-weighed *at the same rate* regained 4lb (1.8kg).
- Those who self-weighed *more* regained 2lb (0.9kg).

'Consistent self-weighing may help individuals maintain their successful weight loss by allowing them to catch weight gains before they escalate, and make behavior changes to prevent additional weight gain,' concluded the researchers in *Obesity*.

That's certainly my experience and my co-author Bill's also. When I was cutting back on calories to lose weight after my pregnancy, I found that self-weighing helped me cheat less. I'd think, 'Yes, I want that extra scoop of ice cream, but I have to face the scales tomorrow!' Bill is also a big fan of daily self-weighing, saying it's a big reason why he still weighs what he weighed at university. When the numbers on his scales start to go up, he makes sure his calorie intake goes down. In his role as a health coach, he counsels his clients to do the same.

***Daily weighing is valuable.*** In another study, researchers at the University of Minnesota tracked more than 3000 people over two years – some in a weight-loss programme and some in a weight-maintenance programme. Those who self-weighed the most during those two years had the *largest weight loss* in the weight-loss programme, and the *smallest weight gain* in the maintenance programme.[5]

'Daily weighing is valuable to individuals trying to lose weight or prevent weight gain,' wrote the researchers in the *Annals of Behavioral Medicine.* 'Daily self-weighing should be emphasized in clinical and public health messages about weight control.' (That's why I'm emphasising it here!)

*When* should you weigh yourself? Do it at the same time every day, because weight varies during the day. First thing in the morning – before you've had anything to eat or drink – is ideal.

---

### FRED'S STORY: 'THIS DIET HAS BEEN PERFECT FOR ME'

*Weight loss: 2 stone 2lb (13.6kg)*

'The Every-Other-Day Diet has been perfect for me,' said Fred Lang, a marketing consultant in Chicago. 'When I'm not on a diet, I normally skip breakfast, and eat a late lunch and a late dinner. So when I heard about Diet Day and Feast Day, the pattern of eating seemed a perfect match with my lifestyle. And it was. I found it very easy to have

*(continued)*

one meal on Diet Day, and then to just relax and eat any-thing I wanted to on Feast Day. On Diet Day, I made sure to drink plenty of water, which helped with hunger. I also drank diet fizzy drinks, chewed gum and had the occasional cup of coffee – all of which have zero calories. I ate one meal – usually a Lean Cuisine ready meal, which was pretty good – and I had a nice snack later in the day. Plus, I knew that however hungry I felt, I would be eating plenty tomorrow.

'Mind you, I didn't have a ton of weight to lose – I'm 5'10" (1.8m) and weighed 13 stone 8lb (86.2kg). But after 12 weeks of EOD dieting I'd lost *all* my extra weight. I'd shed 2 stone 2lb (13.6kg). I can tell you, both me *and* my wife are really happy about that!'

### Tip 2: Eat Lunch or Dinner (but Not Breakfast)

All the participants in my studies on the Every-Other-Day Diet have eaten *lunch* as their Diet Day meal. It's not that I think eating at noon is somehow crucial to losing weight. Rather, using the same Diet Day meal from study to study has allowed me to compare the results of all my various studies, instead of introducing another scientific variable (mealtime) that would make those comparisons more problematic.

If you want to match the methodology of my studies – if you want the highest level of confidence that the pattern of eating you're using is the same pattern scientifically shown to produce steady, significant weight loss – then eat *lunch* on Diet Day.

However, it's quite likely that the success of EOD diet-ing isn't tied to eating lunch. It's tied to a modified fast on

Diet Day and unlimited eating on Feast Day. So if you prefer to eat *dinner* on Diet Day – enjoying dinnertime with your spouse, family, or friends – go right ahead. But I do strongly advise against eating *breakfast* as your main meal on Diet Day, because you may find yourself so hungry by dinnertime that you won't be able to limit yourself to 500 calories for the day. I'm currently conducting a study using lunch *or* dinner as the meal on Diet Day, to see if people eating a lunch-only or dinner-only pattern have the same level of weight loss. Once again, stay tuned!

### Tip 3: Count Your Calories – Not!

One of the wonderful features of the Every-Other-Day Diet is that it's incredibly easy to follow: all you do is eat 500 calories on Diet Day and whatever you want on Feast Day. I've never talked to a single person who really likes calorie counting, even with the new smartphone apps that make the process a little easier, like Lose It! or MyFitness Pal.

Counting calories makes it seem like a calculator is a utensil you have to use at every meal, like mealtime is a contest where you're both competitor and scorekeeper, and you're always about to be (and feel) defeated. In short, it's an annoying mealtime chore you'd rather not do. You want to *enjoy* food, not tabulate it.

Well, the recipes and guidance in this book guarantee that you'll never have to do any complex calorie counting while you're on the Every-Other-Day Diet. Because we've done all the counting for you, in advance.

There are typically two times you take in calories on Diet Day: at your lunch or dinner (about 400 calories), and when you eat your snack (about 100 calories). And there are two ways you can go about your Diet Day meals.

You can make your own food, in which case the recipes in chapter 4 will be hugely helpful. It provides 28 days of 400-calorie lunches, 28 days of 400-calorie dinners, and 28 days of 100-calorie snacks – and those 84 recipes can provide *months* of easy Diet Days.

Say, for example, that your New Year's resolution is to lose 1 stone 6lb (9.1kg), and you start the Every-Other-Day Diet on 2 January. In January, you'll have 15 Diet Days; in February, you'll have 14. If you choose lunch as your Diet Day meal, the lunch recipes in chapter 4 will guide you through two months of dieting. If you decide to switch to dinner for Diet Days in March and April, the recipes will guide you through nearly two more months of Diet Days.

In other words, there are enough recipes in chapter 4 for nearly *four months* of Diet Days, without ever having to count a single calorie or use the same recipe twice. And because those recipes are simple (none of them has more than seven ingredients), speedy (cooking and preparation times are always under 30 minutes) and tasty, you're in for a couple of months of simple (and even fun) Diet Days.

Or you can always opt to microwave a ready meal (see p. 93). Many of the meals are twenty-first-century wonders of culinary ingenuity, delivering maximum flavour and nutrition. They're also perfect for super-easy EOD dieting, since the labels tell you exactly how many calories they contain. On p. 94, we've listed some brands that offer 400 calories or less.

Many participants in my studies prefer the ease and simplicity of using ready meals on Diet Day, and you might feel the same way. You won't have to think twice (or even once) about calories, and preparation takes hardly any time at all.

### Tip 4: Make a Plan for the Day – and Stick with It

What's the biggest mistake my study participants made on Diet Day? Not knowing *exactly* what they were going to eat when mealtime rolled around. Because if you're hungry, you're likely to eat more than 500 calories.

There's an easy way to avoid that mistake: choose your lunch or dinner (and snack) for Diet Day the *night before* and rest easy that you'll have a very successful Diet Day tomorrow.

### Tip 5: Don't Eat Mini-Meals

Over my years of research into EOD dieting, I've been asked by many study participants if they could divide the calories of their Diet Day meal into several low-calorie mini-meals. That way, they reasoned, they could eat throughout the day and feel less hungry. My answer is always *no*. And I have a very good reason for saying no: I want my study participants to actually lose weight!

The problem with eating mini-meals on Diet Day – for example, three 150-calorie meals – is that most of us tend to underestimate calories. What you *think* is 150 calories is probably 200, 250 or more. So instead of eating the 400-calorie Diet Day meal and a 100-calorie Diet Day snack, you might eat three mini-meals of 200, 250 or 300 calories, eat a lot more than 500 calories on Diet Day and slow the pace and amount of weight loss. But if you eat only one meal a day, you have only one opportunity to miscalculate calories.

And if you do err once a day – maybe consuming 100 excess calories – it's not such a big deal.

However, there's an exception to this rule. When you prepare and eat a lunch or dinner recipe from chapter 4, or a ready meal, you know the *exact* amount of calories you're consuming because we've totalled the calories in the recipe, or they're right there on the label of your chosen meal. So feel free to eat the meal any way you like: all at once; half for lunch and half for dinner; or even in thirds. I don't think this strategy is ideal, because it doesn't reflect what worked in my studies. But if you're absolutely certain your intake is under 500 calories, you're still on the Every-Other-Day Diet.

## PROTEIN PACKS A PUNCH

Protein is a powerful tool to fight off hunger and keep you feeling full longer. Researchers at the University of Missouri divided 27 overweight men on a calorie-restricted diet into high- or normal-protein groups. The high-protein group felt *twice* as full during the day as the normal-protein group. 'These data support the consumption of high protein intake, but not greater eating frequency, for improved appetite control and satiety [fullness] ... during calorie restriction-induced weight loss,' the researchers concluded.[6]

In a similar study from researchers at the University of Kansas Medical Center, also published in *Obesity*, 13 obese people ate either three or six meals a day, and the meals were either normal or high protein.[7] And once again, eating more frequently didn't reduce the participants' hunger –

but eating protein did. In fact, eating six meals a day led to 'lower daily fullness'; those who ate *more* frequently felt *more* hungry throughout the day.

**Bottom line:** protein is crucial for helping you feel full and staving off hunger. The hunger-taming power of protein is why many of the recipes in chapter 4, like the Turkey and Avocado Sandwich, and many ready meals have plenty of protein.

*A final note:* don't look to protein bars to mute your appetite. Not only are they typically too high in calories for the Every-Other-Day Diet, but they're often artificially sweetened, which can stimulate appetite. You'll read more about the downsides of artificial sweeteners later in this chapter.

### PAUL'S STORY: 'I FOUND ALTERNATE-DAY FASTING INCREDIBLY EASY TO DO'

*Weight loss: 3 stone 7lb (22.2kg)*

Paul Gower is a 52-year-old in the Fire Safety Department in Malvern, Worcestershire. On Diet Day, he limits his intake to several cups of beef broth, water, four or five cups of coffee, and some raw vegetables, like celery sticks. 'If I eat more than that I find it quite difficult to stop eating,' he told us. But that approach to Diet Day has definitely worked for him. In August 2012, when he started every-other-day dieting, the 5'11" (1.8m) Gower weighed 16 stone 7lb (104.8kg). After a year on the diet, he weighs 13 stone (82.6kg).

*(continued)*

'I found alternate-day fasting incredibly easy to do,' he said. 'The hardest part of the diet is that I do the majority of cooking for my family – I've always cooked and I love to cook. In the early days, I would serve the meal and walk away. Now, I just sit with them and drink my beef broth and eat my celery sticks, and I can cope with it.'

In fact, Diet Days are so easy he barely thinks about them. 'I'm hardly aware of them, they're so much a part of my routine,' he said. 'And I know that I can always eat whatever I want tomorrow – and I do! I've tried many other diets over the years and this is the one that works for me.'

### Tip 6: Don't Skimp on the Fat

Most diets require you to change not only the *amount* of food you're eating, but also the *type* of food. If you're on a Paleo Diet, you can't eat grains, beans or dairy products. If you're on Atkins, you cut carbs. With a plant-based or vegan diet, red meat, fish, dairy and eggs are forbidden. If you're on the Ornish Diet, you restrict fat. If you've decided to hang out in The Zone, you juggle macronutrients, carefully calibrating every meal to include 40 per cent 'good' carbs, 30 per cent fat and 30 per cent protein. And the latest fashion in dieting – reflected in plans like the 17-Day Diet and the Dukan Diet – restricts foods in complex stages, phases and cycles that require a complete change in eating habits every few weeks.

The Every-Other-Day Diet *doesn't* make complicated dietary demands. On Diet Day, you can stick with your current pattern of eating, whatever it is. You don't have to restock your fridge and larder and eat in ways you've never eaten before. Diet Day is about eating fewer *calories* – not some strange mix of macronutrients, or a confusing menu of 'allowed' and 'forbidden' foods.

***Bottom line:*** you can eat anything you want on Diet Day – as long as you eat only 500 calories. And by anything, I mean *anything* – including high-fat foods.

I don't like to see EOD dieters suffer from the problem my co-author Bill and I have dubbed *lipidophobia*: fear of dietary fat. In fact, I'd like to *encourage* you to eat high-fat foods on Diet Day. I know that sounds like weight-loss heresy. But it's the *proven* approach to maximising success on the EOD diet. You'll recall from chapter 1, some of my studies have explored whether eating high- or low-fat food on Diet Day plays any role in how much weight you lose. In one of those studies, I divided participants into two groups: one group ate high-fat foods on Diet Day and the other ate low-fat foods. Those on the high-fat diet (45 per cent fat, 15 per cent protein, 40 per cent carbohydrates) had the following results:

- They lost 17 per cent more weight.
- They lost 32 per cent more body fat.
- They had an 8 per cent increase in muscle (lean body mass), while the low-fat group had no increase.

I had a theory about the pound-shedding, fat-shedding power of high fat: I thought the low-fat group felt deprived and cheated on Diet Day. And when my colleagues and I analysed the data, we found out that was the case; the people eating low-fat foods on Diet Day cheated nearly *twice* as often as those eating high-fat foods.

So go ahead and enjoy high-fat foods – both on Diet Day and on Feast Day. They're delicious and satisfying and, as research suggests, even good for you! Below are some examples of high-fat foods and their benefits.

***More fish oil, longer life.*** A study from researchers at the Harvard School of Public Health found that older people with high blood levels of omega-3 fatty acids – the DHA (docosahexaenoic acid) and EPA (eicosapentaenoic acid) primarily found in fish oil – had a 27 per cent lower risk of death from any cause, mostly because fewer of them died from heart disease, which kills so many people.[8] In fact, people with the highest blood levels of omega-3 fats at age 65 lived an average of 2.2 years longer than people with the lowest levels. Yet many of the adherents of low-fat, plant-based diets specifically tell you *not* to eat EPA- and DHA-rich fatty fish.

***Olive oil and nuts – two high-fat foods – prevent heart attack and stroke.*** In a study published in the *New England Journal of Medicine*, Spanish researchers divided more than 7000 people at high risk for heart disease into three groups: two groups ate a Mediterranean diet rich in either olive oil or nuts. The fat-rich diets lowered the risk of heart attack, stroke and death from heart disease by 30 per cent compared to a low-fat diet – a benefit so impressive the researchers stopped the study because they couldn't ethically keep the third group on a diet that didn't include high-fat foods.[9]

***Saturated fat doesn't cause heart disease.*** Saturated

fat is found mainly in meat and dairy products, and we've been told again and again that it trashes our arteries, triggering heart attack and stroke and that everybody should eat less. Is that good advice? Not according to a study from scientists at the Oakland Research Institute in California, published in the *American Journal of Clinical Nutrition*.[10] The researchers analysed data from 21 other studies, involving more than 340,000 people. They found 'no significant evidence for concluding that dietary saturated fat is associated with increased risk of coronary heart disease or cardiovascular disease.'

On a smaller scale, several of my studies have shown that people who ate high-fat foods on Diet Day had improvements in their risk factors for cardiovascular disease that matched the improvements in people who ate low-fat foods. In other words, high-fat wasn't hurting them, but weight loss was helping them!

It's high time we stopped being afraid of high-fat foods; that's why they're an enjoyable element of the Every-Other-Day Diet.

---

### GERD'S STORY: 'I'M 51 YEARS OLD – BUT I FEEL LIKE I'M 30'

*Weight loss: 1 stone 7lb (9.5kg)*

At 6'3" (1.9m), 51-year-old Gerd Eichele can still carry his weight quite well. 'I'm a big guy, with big bones,' he told us. But a couple of years ago he realised he was carrying a little too much weight. 'A friend of mine took my picture and when I saw it I was shocked. I thought, "Whoa, look at that gut!"'

*(continued)*

Gerd started on a programme of alternate-day fasting in September 2011. He kept his caloric intake on Diet Day at around 750 calories, eating two very low-calorie meals a day and one snack. A breakfast would typically be a medium-sized bowl of porridge, a boiled egg and a glass of orange juice. He would snack on an apple during the day and have a bag of quick-cook steamed vegetables for dinner. When he started every-other-day fasting he weighed 17 stone 1lb (108.4kg). Today he weighs 15 stone 8lb (98.9kg).

'A lot of people started commenting on my weight – even my in-laws. Alternate-day fasting was a little tough at first,' he said. 'But once I got into the swing of it, it was easy. What surprises me the most is that when I wake up in the morning after a day of fasting I'm not really all that hungry.'

Gerd attributes his weight loss not only to every-other-day dieting, but to drinking *lots* of water, which helps him feel full during the day. 'I drink a litre [1³/₄ pints] of water right after I get up in the morning, and continue to drink water throughout the day,' he said.

His third weight-loss secret, along with every-other-day dieting and water: regular exercise. 'I walk about three miles a day, and six or seven miles once a week,' he said. 'I listen to music or podcasts while I walk, and the time really flies by. This combination – every-other-day fasting, lots of water, and regular exercise – really hits the mark.'

Gerd feels like he could lose a few more pounds and 'discover' his abs, which are still covered up by a bit of fat. 'I'm sure that with alternate-day fasting, drinking plenty of water, and regular exercise I'll reach that goal, too.'

## Tip 7: If You're Eating Out on Diet Day, Check the Menu Before You Go!

Of course, at some point, you're going to find yourself eating out on Diet Day, which is a little bit like tiptoeing through a minefield where the mines are calories that could blow up your diet. It's risky! For that reason, I strongly recommend you try to avoid it as much as possible, but if you do go, here is my top tip: plan ahead.

**Many restaurants now offer calorie counts online or even on the menu. These include:**

- Fast-food restaurants like McDonald's, Burger King and KFC
- The Real Greek, Leon, Café Rouge, Prezzo and Zizzi
- Pizza Hut, Dominos
- Harvester or Wetherspoons
- Nandos
- Carluccios
- Yo Sushi
- Sandwich/coffee bars such as those of main supermarkets, or Pret A Manger, Subway or Starbucks and Costa

Before you go out, go online and check the calorie counts of items on the menu that you like, to see if they match up with the calorie limit of Diet Day. You could also try a website which puts a range of restaurant meals all on one site such as www.weightlossresources.co.uk or a phone app such as Nutracheck.

Some restaurants such as Café Rouge, Subway, Frankie

and Benny's, Pizza Express or Pizza Hut also offer a range of 'Healthier Choices' with, for example, some subs or pizzas under 500 calories.

You can assume that just about everything else on the menu – *including the starters* – is over 500 calories. Way over.

My essential message is this: *know* the calories in any dish you're ordering by first finding out the calorie level online (although some places do now post calorie content on the menu board as well). And *don't* order any dish or meal if you're guessing its calorie level. Chances are, you're guessing wrong.

When it comes to fast-food restaurants the number of meals that can work on Diet Day may surprise you. For example, McDonald's claims that 80 per cent of the items on its menu are under 400 calories – a fit for Diet Day. And that's true. A Filet-O-Fish is 335 calories. A Cheeseburger is 295 calories. Six Chicken McNuggets are 250 calories. And a grilled chicken and bacon salad (without dressing) is 190 calories.

So, if you're determined to eat at McDonald's on Diet Day (or any other fast-food restaurant), you McCan! Just go online *first*, work out what you want, check the calories – and stick to your calorie-smart choices when you're at the restaurant.

### Tip 8:  Make the Most of Your Snack on Diet Day

The typical Diet Day includes a 400-calorie meal (either lunch or dinner) and a 100-calorie snack. If you eat a Diet Day lunch or dinner that is *less* than 400 calories, you can eat a snack that is *more* than 100 calories. Or if you go for a frozen ready meal that is around 300 calories – and there are many choices out there – you can eat two 100-calorie snacks.

What kind of snack should you eat? In chapter 4, you'll

find delicious recipes for 28 100-calorie snacks, like Frozen Berry lollies, Greek Yogurt Parfait and Chocolate Stack.

When should you have your snack? The participants in my studies have eaten their Diet Day snack at any time: first thing in the morning, mid-morning, mid-afternoon, early evening, before bed – even in the middle of the night! What's best is what's best for *you* – eat your snack when you want it the most and enjoy it the most.

During the first two weeks or so of the EOD Diet – when you may still be feeling hungry on Diet Day – eat your snack at the time you're hungriest. In other words, use it to reduce hunger. After two weeks on the Every-Other-Day Diet, when hunger on Diet Day has pretty much disappeared, eat the snack for enjoyment and energy, at the time of day when you find you're most refreshed and renewed by having something to eat.

Aside from your personal preferences, however, nutritional science provides a few guidelines about the best time of day to snack for weight loss.

***Afternoon is better than mid-morning.*** Researchers at the University of Illinois studied 123 overweight women who were on a one-year weight-loss programme. Those who snacked in the afternoon lost 7 per cent more weight than those who snacked mid-morning, the researchers reported in the *Journal of the American Dietetic Association*.[11]

***Night-time might not be the right time.*** Women who snacked at night burned 12 per cent less fat than people who snacked during the daytime, reported Japanese researchers. 'Eating at night...increases the risk of obesity,' they wrote in the *American Journal of Physiology: Regulatory, Integrative and Comparative Physiology*.[12]

## SCIENTIFIC SURPRISE: SNACKING CAN BE GOOD FOR YOU

We are snacking more than ever: over the past few decades, the percentage of American adults who snack rose from 71 per cent to 97 per cent. We're eating an average of one more snack per day than we used to. The percentage of total daily calories from snacks rose from 18 per cent to 24 per cent. And we're consuming more salty snacks, biscuits, sweets and sugar-sweetened drinks. There are plenty of studies that link snacking – and its added calories – to added pounds. But what you typically don't hear is the *good* news about snacking. For example:

*If you start eating smaller, low-calorie snacks, you quickly adapt to the smaller size and regularly eat smaller snacks.* Researchers at the Center for Human Nutrition at the University of Colorado studied 59 people, testing the effect of eating 100-calorie snacks. They found the individuals quickly adapted to the smaller snacks and stopped eating bigger ones.[13]

Well, you won't find any snack larger than 100 calories in chapter 4, but you'll quickly get used to eating and enjoying these smaller, lower-calorie goodies.

*Snacks improve your diet.* A team of researchers from Auburn University in Alabama noted that snacking has a bad reputation: it's thought to contribute nothing more than empty calories to the diet. But in a five-year study of more than 11,000 adults, they found ('contrary to expectation') that people who snacked scored *higher* on the

Healthy Eating Index. The more people snacked, the more fruits, whole grains and milk products they ate. 'Snacking was associated with a more nutrient-dense diet,' wrote the researchers in the *Journal of the Academy of Nutrition and Dietetics*.[14]

**Senior citizens – start your snacking!** When the researchers at Auburn focused on 2000 people aged 65 and older, they found those who snacked more also had higher intakes of vitamins A, C, E and beta-carotene, and the minerals magnesium and potassium. 'Nutritional benefits obtained from snack food and beverages warrant their inclusion in older adults' diet,' they concluded in the *Journal of the American Dietetic Association*.[15]

**Snacks help you maintain weight loss.** In a study of 257 adults, people who lost weight and maintained it ate 21 per cent more snacks than those who were overweight. 'Two snacks per day may be important in weight loss maintenance,' wrote the researchers in the *Journal of the American Dietetic Association*.[16]

**Bottom line:** develop a knack for snacks!

## THE FOUR BEST WAYS TO EASE YOUR HUNGER ON DIET DAY

My research shows that people feel hungry on Diet Day for about the first two to three weeks of the Every-Other-Day Diet, and then hunger pretty much disappears. How do you deal with your hunger on Diet Day during those first few weeks? EOD dieters say a couple of strategies work best.

### 1. Drink a Glass (or Two) of Water

The people in my studies consistently tell me that when they're hungry on Diet Day, nothing works as well to mute their appetite as drinking a glass (or two) of water. They drink 8, 10, 12 or 16 fluid ounces (0.2 – 0.45 litres), and in just a few minutes their hunger level noticeably declines.

These EOD dieters are finding out for themselves what scientists have been discovering over the past couple of years: study after study is showing the power of water to diminish appetite.

Here are some of the recent findings supporting the power of a glass of water to wash away Diet Day discomfort and help you shed pounds.

***Drink water before a meal and feel fuller and less hungry.*** Researchers at Virginia Tech studied 50 people, dividing them into two groups: half drank 17 fluid ounces (0.5 litres) of water 30 minutes before lunch, and half didn't. Those who drank water ate an average of 58 fewer calories at lunchtime and also felt less hungry and more full.[17]

In a similar study from the same researchers, people who drank the same amount of water 30 minutes before breakfast ate 74 fewer calories in the meal.[18]

'Drinking water reduces sensations of hunger and increases satiety, the sensation of feeling full,' says Brenda Davy, PhD, RD, the leader of these studies and an associate professor in the Department of Nutrition, Foods and Exercise at Virginia Tech.

***Drink more water, burn more calories.*** Drinking 17 fluid ounces (0.5 litres) of water triggers the body to increase calorie burning by 24 per cent over the next hour, reported

German researchers in the *Journal of Clinical Endocrinology and Metabolism.*[19]

These researchers aren't just talking about drinking a glass of *cold* water, thereby speeding up metabolism as your body tries to reheat itself. *Any* temperature of drinking water causes an increase in calorie-burning because a glass of water stimulates the sympathetic nervous system, increasing metabolic rate.

***Drink more water, lose more weight.*** Researchers at Virginia Tech studied 40 people: 20 were instructed to drink 16 fluid ounces (0.45 litres) of water before every meal and record their daily water intake; the other 20 didn't pay any extra attention to their daily hydration. After one year, the group that was attentive to water intake lost 87 per cent more weight.[20]

***Bottom line:*** hydrate! Drink 16 fluid ounces (0.45 litres) of water *whenever* you feel hungry, 30 minutes or so before your Diet Day meal and 30 minutes or so before your Diet Day snack. Another good strategy: carry a water bottle with you and drink as often as possible throughout the day.

---

### SICK OF PLAIN WATER? INFUSE!

Many of the participants in my studies said they got tired of drinking plain water and solved the problem by drinking carbonated or soda water or by adding a squeeze of lemon or lime. But there's another way to spruce up a plain glass of water, turning it into a delicious, delicately flavoured drink: infusion.

You can buy an 'infusion pitcher' for about £14–25 on Amazon or other online retailers. Essentially, it's a big water

*(continued)*

jug with a rod or chamber in the middle, into which you can put, well, just about *anything* you like. The infusing ingredient stays in the chamber and flavours the water. Try lemon, orange and/or grapefruit slices, berries or cherries, cucumbers and lemongrass (the combo used in many spas) or watermelon and kiwi. Or use herbs like mint, rosemary, lavender or camomile to make a delicious iced tea. Really, any combination of fruits, herbs or refreshing vegetables you'd like to try. And you can use any type of water – plain, carbonated or soda. The infusion ingredients will stay fresh for ten days, as long as you refrigerate the jug. Just refill and drink up!

## 2. Skip the Diet Soda and Avoid Artificial Sweeteners – They Might Make You *Hungrier*

Because water is so effective at reducing hunger and aiding weight loss, you might think *any* no-calorie beverage can do the same, like no-calorie diet fizzy drinks, diet energy drinks and diet sports drinks. These artificially sweetened products can be a good strategy for some people, but I'm not a big fan of drinking them on Diet Day, for a few reasons:

***More diet fizzy drinks result in more eating.*** A study in the journal *Appetite* showed that people who drink two or more artificially sweetened drinks per day have a *harder* time controlling their appetite and have a tendency to overeat.[21] And scientists think they may know why. Researchers in the Department of Psychiatry at Yale University School of Medicine scanned the brains of 26 people while they used an artificial sweetener and found that being exposed to a sweet taste *without* ingesting any calories may cause the brain to generate cravings for more sweet foods! I'm not surprised by these results. In my studies, about 4 out of 5 participants get a surge of hunger after drinking a diet fizzy drink.

**Drinking three diet fizzy drinks a day doubles your risk of obesity.** In a seven-year study from the University of Texas Health Science Center involving more than 3600 people, those who drank three or more artificially sweetened beverages per day were nearly *twice* as likely to become overweight or obese. 'These findings raise the question,' wrote the researchers in *Obesity*, whether artificially sweetened beverages 'might be fueling – rather than fighting – our escalating obesity epidemic.'[22]

**Artificial sweeteners can lead to disease.** Other studies link diet fizzy drinks to disease; compared to people who don't drink them, those who do had:

- *a 16 per cent higher risk of stroke*, per fizzy drink, per day. (In other words, if you regularly drink two per day, your risk is 32 per cent higher.[23])
- *a 42 per cent higher risk of leukaemia,* per fizzy drink per day.[24]
- *a 67 per cent higher risk for type-2 diabetes*, from daily consumption of one or more diet fizzy drinks. Research published in *Diabetes Care* shows that they stimulate the release of GLP-1 (glucagon-like peptide 1), a compound linked to the development of type-2 diabetes.[25]
- *a 220 per cent higher risk for chronic kidney disease* for people consuming two or more diet fizzy drinks per day.[26]

So my advice is to limit artificial sweeteners wherever you can. However, if occasionally you want a drink with a low-calorie sweetener, I recommend any of those available on the market such as Hermestas, Sweetex, Canderel or a new pleasant-tasting sweetener stevia (made from the leaves of the stevia plant, a sweet-tasting herb in the chrysanthemum family, which is sold in the UK as Truvia). These have all received approval as safe for human use by the European Food Safety Authority (EFSA).

Why don't we recommend aspartame or sucralose (Splenda)? Because those are the two sweeteners used in most diet fizzy drinks – drinks that are increasingly linked to health problems, as we just discussed. As we were writing this book, a new study in *Diabetes Care* from researchers at the University of Washington in Seattle showed that ingesting Splenda spiked blood sugar and insulin levels in obese people.[27]

## CAN YOU DRINK ALCOHOL ON DIET DAY?

For many of us, drinking a beer, a glass of wine or spirits is one of the happy pleasures of daily life - it refreshes, relaxes and enhances your enjoyment of social time with family and friends. Research also shows that moderate drinking - no more than 3–4 units a day for men and 2–3 units a day for women - can reduce the risk of heart disease. (One drink is 5 ounces of wine, 12 ounces of beer, or 1½ ounces of distilled spirits, such as whisky or vodka.)

If you enjoy alcohol in moderation, there's no need to stop on the Every-Other-Day Diet. Like any other food or beverage, there's no limit to alcohol intake on Feast Day, other than common sense.

But what about Diet Day? Well, think carefully before imbibing. Because along with that pleasant buzz, alcohol can deliver a lot of calories.

For example, if you down a large margarita, you're also downing nearly 300 calories – 60 per cent of your Diet Day quota!

Not all drinks are super-caloric, of course. Red wine delivers 110 calories; beer, 150 to 200. There are ultra-light beers that deliver less than 100 calories. And you don't have to down an entire drink: for example, if you limit yourself to a small glass of white wine, it's about 90 calories.

But my general recommendation for drinking alcohol on Diet Day is simple: just say no. It's too high in calories. And because it affects your judgment and can be a typical meal-time accompaniment, it's too easy to decide to have a second drink. Before you know it, Diet Day has turned into eat, drink and be merry day.

If you do decide to have a drink on Diet Day, have only one, and treat it as your snack for the day, ensuring that it fits in with the calorie level of your lunch or dinner. So if your main meal is 350 calories, you could accompany it with a 150-calorie beer.

*(continued)*

> **Bottom line:** if you'd like to 'snack' on an alcoholic drink on Diet Day, go ahead. But be aware of the calories it contains, and don't overdo it.

### 3. A Cup of Coffee or Tea a Day Can Keep the Hunger Away

Both black coffee and tea are good ways to cut hunger without adding calories. When overweight and obese people drank a cup of strong coffee with breakfast, they ate less at lunch and throughout the day, reported researchers in *Obesity*.[28]

***More coffee, more weight loss.*** In a 12-year study of nearly 58,000 people, those who increased their coffee consumption during the study gained less weight, reported researchers from the Harvard School of Public Health.[29] When researchers analysed 11 studies on green tea and dieting, they similarly found that people who drank tea lost up to 3.3lb (1.5kg) more than those who didn't.

***Catechins and caffeine: low hunger, high fullness.*** Bill's book *The Natural Fat-Loss Pharmacy* devotes an entire chapter to the appetite-taming, fat-fighting power of tea – black, green and white (oolong) tea – with green tea leading the way. The secret ingredient in tea? It's *catechins*: powerful plant compounds with a wide range of health-giving effects, like lowering the risk of heart disease and cancer. A drink containing green tea catechins and caffeine (along with fibre) 'created the lowest hunger and the highest fullness ratings' and the lowest energy [calorie] intake at the next meal,' reported researchers in the journal *Appetite*.[30]

***Tea trims body fat.*** Habitual tea drinkers (15 fluid ounces (426ml) daily) have 20 per cent less body fat than people who don't drink tea, according to a study in *Obesity Research.*

***Catechins help people burn more calories and fat.*** Drinking a catechin-rich tea throughout the day triggered 12 per cent more fat-burning than drinking water, according to a study in the *Journal of Nutrition.* In another study, obese dieters who took a supplement with green tea catechins burned 43 more calories per day – and lost 7.3lb (3.3kg) more after 12 weeks, compared to dieters who didn't take the green tea supplement.

***Catechins help you do better with weight maintenance.*** Getting more green tea catechins in the diet helped people 'significantly maintain body weight after a period of weight loss,' reported Dutch researchers in the *International Journal of Obesity.*[31]

***Bottom line:*** coffee and/or tea, particularly green tea, are great choices for no-calorie drinks on Diet Day. And they're good for you, too. Recent studies link regular coffee drinking to a wide range of health benefits, including less risk of type-2 diabetes, gallbladder disease, Alzheimer's, Parkinson's and liver cancer. One 13-year study of more than 52,000 people showed that regular coffee drinkers even had lower 'all-cause mortality' – during the study compared to people who didn't drink coffee.[32]

Green tea also has a positive effect on health: studies link green tea and its catechins to lower risk for heart disease, and lower risk for many types of cancer, type-2 diabetes, and Alzheimer's disease.

But take care with the milk and sugar. If you want to add a little to your coffee or tea, go ahead, but you'll have to count calories. For example, a tablespoon of skimmed milk has 6 calories; a tablespoon of full-fat milk has 20; and a tablespoon of semi-skimmed, 9. A packet of sugar adds 11 calories. If you have four cups of coffee on Diet Day with a touch of full-fat milk and a packet of sugar, you're adding 80 calories – in effect, your four cups of coffee have become your daily snack.

### 4. Chew Up Your Hunger with Sugar-Free Gum

One of the best ways to stave off hunger on Diet Day, say my study participants, is to *chew gum*. It keeps your mouth busy. And it seems to 'fool' your body into thinking you're eating something. There are some studies about the effects of gum chewing:

***People feel less hungry and burn more calories.*** In his book *Breakthroughs in Natural Healing 2011*, Bill reported on two studies showing that chewing sugar-free gum can help you feel less hungry, so you eat fewer calories and burn more. The first study was conducted by Kathleen Melanson, PhD, RD, an associate professor of nutrition and food science at the University of Rhode Island. The 35 participants in the two-day study chewed sugar-free gum on only one of the two days in three 20-minute sessions of 'relaxed, natural' chewing: one session before breakfast and two between breakfast and lunch. The results? On the day of gum-chewing, participants felt less hungry, consumed an average of 68 fewer calories at lunch and didn't consume more calories later in the day. The participants also burned about 5 per cent more calories during the gum-chewing sessions. And they felt more upbeat on the day they chewed gum: they had more energy, and it seemed to take less energy to accomplish tasks.

'Gum-chewing may be a useful addition to a weight-management programme,' concluded Dr Melanson, who reported her research at an annual meeting of the Obesity Society. 'Gum-chewing might cut hunger and calorie intake in two ways,' Dr Melanson told Bill. 'The sensations in the mouth might send "I'm full" signals to the brain's appetite centre. And nerves in the muscles of the jaw that are stimulated by gum-chewing might send those signals, too.

'If you're attempting to lose weight, give gum-chewing a try to see if it works to help you feel less hungry and cut calories,' she continued. 'Use sugar-free gum as one tool in your weight-loss toolbox.'

***Seven smart times to chew gum.*** Another study on gum-chewing in overweight people was reported at the same meeting by Leah Whigham, PhD, a nutrition scientist at the government's Grand Forks Human Nutrition Research Center in North Dakota.

Dr Whigham and her colleagues found that overweight people who typically needed a lot of 'cognitive restraint' in order to control their eating habits – people who had to remind themselves again and again *not* to eat, so they wouldn't mindlessly snack or eat when they weren't hungry – ate fewer daily calories when they chewed gum six times a day for 15 minutes each time.

Dr Whigham suggests chewing sugar-free gum at the following times:

- when you're craving a high-calorie snack
- when watching TV, instead of snacking
- for 15 minutes immediately after lunch or dinner
- when you go out to eat, while waiting for the main course
- in 'high-risk' situations for overeating, such as at parties, weddings, sporting events or the cinema
- when you're bored, since boredom is often a trigger for eating and overeating
- when you're stressed, since stress is also a trigger.

***More gum-chewing, less hunger, less appetite and fewer craving for sweets.*** In a four-day study, researchers in the UK asked 60 people to eat lunch and then rate their hunger, appetite and craving for sweet and salty snacks every hour for three hours. On two days of the study, the participants chewed gum for 15 minutes for each of the three hours, totalling 45 minutes. On the other two days, they didn't chew gum. 'Chewing gum for at least 45 minutes significantly suppressed hunger, appetite and craving for snacks and promoted fullness,' wrote the researchers in *Appetite*.[33] 'This study', they continued, demonstrated the 'benefit of chewing gum ... to those seeking an aid to appetite control.'

***More chewing, less stress.*** Chewing gum can also help you resist stress. In a study conducted by researchers in the UK, people who chewed gum daily for two weeks had less 'perceived stress' and felt they could get more work done, compared to people who didn't chew gum.[34]

In a similar study, in *Current Medical Research and Opinion*, people said that stressful emotions (not feeling relaxed, feeling tense) increased when they *didn't* chew gum.[35]

And in a study by Australian researchers, chewing gum reduced anxiety and stress, reduced the production of the stress hormone cortisol and increased alertness.[36]

## EXERCISE IS OK ON DIET DAY IF YOU EXERCISE *BEFORE* A MEAL

As you read in chapter 1, I've conducted studies to determine if people could exercise comfortably on the EOD Diet. The results: study participants exercised without problems, whether they worked out on Diet Day, Feast Day or on both. But there was one caveat: exercising late in the day on Diet Day wasn't a good idea. People who did so felt ravenous after their workout, but they'd already consumed 400 of their 500 daily calories, or all 500.

There are three good times to exercise on Diet Day. They are:

- first thing in the morning, perhaps eating your 100-calorie snack straight afterward; or
- immediately before lunch; or
- immediately before dinner, if you choose dinner as your Diet Day meal.

In other words, exercise *before* a meal.

You'll find much more about EOD dieting and exercise in chapter 5, 'Every-Other-Day Dieting and Exercise'.

## SARAH'S STORY: 'I WAS A SIZE 22 AND NOW I'M A 16'

*Weight loss: 2 stone 8lb (16.3kg)*

Sarah is a nurse who works at the Veterans Administration hospital near the University of Illinois-Chicago, where she saw a leaflet recruiting people for a weight-loss study using alternate-day modified fasting. 'I needed to lose weight, and I thought participating in the study would be a great way to do it,' she said.

And lose weight she did. At 5'2" (1.6m) tall, Sarah started the diet weighing 14 stone 11lb (93.9kg), and now she weighs 12 stone 3lb (77.6kg).

'I've gone down six dress sizes!' she exclaimed. 'And my cholesterol dropped, too – from slightly over 200 to 180. The first two weeks of the Every-Other-Day Diet were kind of rough, because of the hunger on Diet Day, but that went away, and every-other-day dieting became my life. And it was easy. For example, if I knew a special occasion was coming up on a Diet Day, I'd just flip-flop a Feast Day and a Diet Day. The key was *planning*.

'I also found that I ate much less on Feast Day than I thought I would. After a few weeks on the diet, it seemed like I was satisfied more quickly by my Feast Day meals, and I almost never overate.'

Sarah also added exercise to her regime. 'Along with the EOD Diet, I do aqua-aerobics, kick-boxing, jogging, walking – anything to help me burn more calories and look thinner,' she said. 'I also weigh myself regularly, to make sure I'm not gaining the weight back.'

## DON'T WORRY ABOUT CHEATING NOW AND THEN

Let's face it: you're probably going to cheat now and then. You're only human!

So, don't worry about it! The participants in my studies who lose the most weight are 'adherent' on Diet Day (that is, they don't cheat) on eight or nine days out of ten. In other words, they occasionally cheat – and it doesn't matter. After all, sometimes your Diet Day is going to fall on a special occasion, like Christmas or New Year, a birthday party or another time when you want to join in the fun.

So go ahead and do it! For example, if Diet Day falls on Christmas Day, eat Christmas dinner, even if the day before was a Feast Day. The day *after* can be Diet Day instead.

It's fine if once or twice a month Diet Day doesn't work out. If you eat 500 calories on most Diet Days, you *will* lose weight. The trick is, if you go off the EOD Diet, just go back on it again the next Diet Day. Cheat on Tuesday; get back on the diet on Thursday. Another possible strategy: if you blow it on Diet Day, relax, turn it into Feast Day, and do Diet Day the next day. But ...

*Don't* beat yourself up – you're just hurting yourself.

*Don't* feel like a failure – you're on the scientifically-proven way to weight-loss success!

*Don't* binge if you go off the diet on Diet Day – because

you can eat whatever you want (and as much as you want) on Feast Day.

*Relax* – and just go back on the diet.

## THE SIMPLEST DIET

The best feature of Diet Day is that it's so *easy*. You're not counting calories or following complex rules – you just eat one low-calorie meal and one snack. There are easy ways to tame Diet Day hunger, which only lasts for the first two weeks or so of the diet, after which you hardly notice it. And maybe the best feature of Diet Day is that it's followed by Feast Day, a day of unrestricted eating. Yes, a day of unlimited eating pleasure is actually part of a *diet*. To learn all about Feast Day, just turn the page.

---

### EOD – EASY AS 1-2-3!

1. Follow one simple rule: eat 500 calories on Diet Day and eat whatever you want the next day.
2. Weigh yourself in the morning, make an eating plan for Diet Day and eat a 400-calorie lunch or dinner and a 100-calorie snack.
3. Drink water, coffee and/or tea, chew sugar-free gum and use other easy methods to mute hunger on Diet Day.

---

CHAPTER 3

# Feast Day

*Eat all you want and anything you want - and keep losing weight!*

This is the shortest chapter in the book, and for good reason: there's only one easy-to-follow 'rule' on Feast Day (the day that alternates with the 500-calorie modified fast of Diet Day). **Eat all the food you want, and eat any kind of food you want.**

I know, I know. It's hard to believe that you don't have to deprive yourself every day while dieting and that you can *still* lose weight; that a diet can include days on which you eat as much food as you want and whatever foods you want and you *still* lose weight. It probably goes against everything you've ever been told about dieting and everything you've ever done while on a diet.

Well, it was also hard to believe for some of my study participants. As veterans of many diets – and many days of diet-based deprivation and denial – they couldn't imagine how they could possibly lose weight while following the Feast Day 'rule' every other day.

And because they so badly wanted to lose weight, many of them kept on restricting their food choices on Feast Day – until we talked them out of it! But once they got used to alternating a day of modified fasting with a day of unlimited eating, they loved it. Feast Day was a *relief* from restriction. And Feast Day made the 500 calories of Diet Day easy, because participants knew they could always eat their favourite foods the next day. Any food. In any quantity. At any time.

## EOD Dieters Rave About Feast Day

Still find it hard to believe that you can eat whatever you want on Feast Day and lose weight? Then listen to what some veteran EOD dieters – people who have lost anywhere from 1 stone 2lb (7.3kg) to 3 stone 7lb (22.2kg) – have to say about it:

*I always enjoy Feast Day.* 'One day fasting and one day feasting is a wonderful pattern. Some days I eat a lot on my Feast Day, and some days I don't, but I always enjoy the day. And my weight continues to go down!' – *Paul, weight loss: 2 stone 13lb (18.6kg)*

*I never feel deprived.* 'On the Every-Other-Day Diet, I can always eat the next day, so I never feel deprived. If I can't have it today, I can have it tomorrow. Knowing that, I can stay on the diet.' – *Susan, weight loss: 3 stone (19.1kg)*

***I stop eating when I feel satisfied and full.*** 'At first, I really had a lot of anticipation about Feast Day, thinking I would just eat as much as I could. But when the day rolled around, I found myself thinking, "Do I really need all that food?" I did eat a little more than normal, of course. But it seemed as if I was satisfied sooner at every meal – that I had learned what feeling *full* is all about, and I could stop eating when I felt full. If it wasn't for the Every-Other-Day Diet, I never would have learned how to do that.' – *Sarah, weight loss: 1 stone 3lb (7.7kg)*

***It's not difficult at all.*** 'I eat heavy one day and light the next, and it's not difficult at all. It's become a habit.' – *Bella, weight loss: 1 stone 11lb (11.3kg)*

***I eat whenever I'm hungry.*** 'On Feast Day, I'm very liberal about what I eat and don't eat. I start with a big, healthy breakfast, and then eat whenever I'm hungry, grazing throughout the day. I love it.' – *Gerd, weight loss: 1 stone 7lb (9.5kg)*

***I look forward to the days I'm not fasting.*** 'I look forward to the days I'm not fasting and can do whatever I want. I don't have to think – "How many calories in this, how many calories in that?" – and that makes the day a whole lot easier.' – *Victoria, weight loss: 1 stone 13lb (12.2kg)*

***I've been on a lot of other diets, and I always get tired of them.*** 'I like this diet because I get to *eat*. I've been on a lot of other diets – like diets where you drink two milkshakes and eat one meal a day – and I always get tired of them because you're basically restricted to the same foods, over and over again.' – *Andrea, weight loss: 1 stone 2lb (7.3kg)*

***I eat what I want.*** 'The Every-Other-Day Diet is very easy to do. I eat what I want on Feast Day, have one well-planned meal on Diet Day – and don't worry about it!' – *Paul, weight loss: 3 stone 7lb (22.2kg)*

Here's what's not hard to believe: Feast Day is the feature of the EOD Diet that study participants like the second best (after losing all the weight they wanted to lose and keeping it off). And EOD dieters were delighted by the biggest surprise of every-other-day dieting: you don't lose control on Feast Day. You don't binge. You don't even eat all that much more. Remember, in my studies, EOD dieters ate only about 10 per cent more calories than normal on Feast Day.

*Do the pound-shedding maths:*

- You eat 25 per cent of your normal calories on Diet Day.
- You eat 110 per cent of your normal calories on Feast Day.
- Your two-day intake is an average of 67.5 per cent of normal calories – 32.5 per cent below normal.
- And that lower level of calories drives steady, safe, *significant* weight loss.

The fact that people don't go into overeating overdrive on Feast Day surprised me, too, at first. But after nearly a decade of research on hundreds of people, I feel confident that alternating a day of modified fasting with a day of unlimited eating *helps* overweight and obese people bring their appetite under control. Let's take a closer look at some of that research.

## THE SURPRISING SCIENCE OF FEAST DAY

In our scientific studies on the EOD Diet, my colleagues and I take one of two approaches to providing food:

1. At the beginning of the study we teach the participants how to eat on Diet Day and Feast Day, and then the participants are on their own; or

2. we supply the participants with pre-packaged, calorie-controlled meals and snacks for both Diet Day and Feast Day.

The first few studies we conducted followed Approach No.2: the food was supplied. But we quickly found out (much to our amazement) that we were supplying *more* food on Feast Day than the study participants could eat.

Specifically, we gave study participants 125 per cent of their normal caloric intake on Feast Day. But they always told us that we were giving them way too much food and they couldn't eat it all.

The same phenomenon is occurring in my three-year, NIH-sponsored study to test weight maintenance after the Every-Other-Day Diet. Once again, the study participants were given pre-packaged, calorie-controlled meals – in this case, 50 per cent of normal calories on Diet Day, and 150 per cent on Feast Day.

Well, it turned out that nobody could eat all their 'assigned' foods on Feast Day. Everybody in the study easily and spontaneously wanted to eat *less* than the 150 per cent. It doesn't seem to make sense, right? After all, experts never tire of telling us that the main reason why people are overweight is the huge portions delivered by restaurants and convenience foods, and the 24/7 availability of food; that when a human being has access to a lot of food, they will *eat* a lot of food. So we imagine that people on the EOD Diet will inevitably pig out on Feast Day. But they don't.

Feast Day isn't a trough. It's a fun, relaxed, and reasonable way to eat. After eating 25 per cent of normal caloric intake on Diet Day, EOD dieters usually eat only 110 per cent of normal calories on Feast Day. Below are my theories about why this happens.

**Metabolic reboot.** The EOD Diet may reset your metabolism – how your body uses food for energy – in ways that science doesn't yet understand but that are profoundly healthy. For example, on most diets you shed 75 per cent fat and 25 per cent muscle. On the EOD Diet, however, you lose about 99 per cent fat and 1 per cent muscle. And if you exercise while on the EOD Diet, you *gain* muscle. That's remarkable. And it's not the only remarkable 'reset' produced by every-other-day dieting.

Not only does the EOD Diet lower LDL cholesterol, it specifically lowers the levels of the hard, dense LDL particles that do the most damage to your arteries. And people on the EOD Diet have an unusually large spike in levels of adiponectin, a hormone that protects your heart. Plus, a growing body of cellular animal and human research shows that every-other-day eating strengthens brain cells. I suspect those remarkable changes extend to appetite.

Every other day, you're allowed to eat all you want. But because you're on the EOD Diet, your body has a better idea: it decides to regulate appetite, so you don't overeat and hurt your health.

**Stomach-shrinking.** The very low-calorie intake of Diet Day may gradually shrink the stomach, reducing appetite.

**No-binge psychology.** The fact that you *can* binge on the Feast Day may *prevent* a binge. When foods are forbidden, you crave them and end up bingeing sooner or later. On the other hand, when foods are allowed, they're not as tempting, and you can take them or leave them.

***Tuning in to true hunger.*** You don't eat until lunch on Diet Day, so you experience *real hunger.* And that's a new experience for the average Westerner, who eats so constantly during the day that he or she almost never experiences the body's *natural hunger cues* – the body letting the brain know when it's time to eat. Instead, most people experience only *emotional hunger cues* – the stress, anger, depression, anxiety and boredom that drive us to eat for emotional comfort rather than physical well-being. On Diet Day, you learn what hunger feels like – and that new-found understanding extends to Feast Day.

Of course, you don't have to understand *why* the EOD Diet works in order to control your appetite; the EOD Diet controls appetite automatically!

## Allison's story: 'This can't be a diet!'

*Weight loss: 7lb (3.2kg)*

Allison P. Davis, an editor at *Elle* magazine, wrote about the Every-Other-Day Diet in the February 2013 issue, in an article entitled 'Halftime Diet'. In the article, she used the terms I use in my scientific papers: *alternate-day fasting* for the EOD Diet; *fast day* for Diet Day; and *feed day* for Feast Day.

Allison had tried WeightWatchers and other diets. But, she wrote, 'Any decision I make to cut back instantly

*(continued)*

activates my instinct to gorge.' What would happen to that 'instinct' on the EOD Diet?

On Diet Days, she wrote, 'it was a comfort just to know that at the stroke of midnight I could have whatever I wanted again. And it was freeing to stop counting calories and making trade-offs. I wasn't swapping points or keeping a diary; I was simply eating.'

But after a Feast Day 'involving mimosas, a fried chicken sandwich, and a side of bacon', she phoned Monica Klempel, PhD, a nutritionist who has helped me conduct many of the studies.

'This can't be a diet!' she shouted over the phone.

'Well, it sounds like you're doing it right,' Dr Klempel replied.

Allison wrote: 'Fasting, Dr Klempel explained, plays a mind game of sorts: most subjects in both of Varady's studies tended to think they were consuming more calories on feed days than they really were. Though that fried chicken seemed unforgivably decadent, I'd eaten only half of it. This was occurring on most feed days: once I got past the initial cravings, the natural desire for fruits and vegetables took over. At the office cafeteria, I'd steer toward the sushi bar rather than the grill. And the scale crept down: I lost a pound and a half the first week; seven by the end of the month.'

After talking with Dr Klempel, Allison talked to a dietitian who was sceptical that the EOD Diet would work long-term. Later, she called me and described the dietitian's doubts. People can and do stay on the diet long-term, I told her –

and the high-fat version of the EOD Diet makes it even more feasible.

She ended her article with this quote from me, and I'd say the same thing today: 'It's really only having to diet half the time. People can really stick to that.'

## REMEMBER: HIGH-FAT IS ON THE FEAST DAY MENU

When I say you can eat *any* type of food you want on Feast Day, I mean *any* type of food – and that includes the high-fat foods found in the typical Western diet. As I discussed in chapters 1 and 2, my studies show that dieters lose *more* weight when they eat high-fat foods on Diet Day and Feast Day. Yes, *more weight.*

For me, these studies confirm the essential principle and practice of the Every-Other-Day Diet: **you don't change *what* you're eating. You change your *pattern* of eating.** You consume 500 calories on Diet Day – eating any type of food. There is no calorie restriction on Feast Day – and you eat any type of food. *And that's it!* The EOD Diet is *simple.* The EOD Diet is *powerful.* Most importantly, the EOD Diet is *effective.*

## ENJOY FEAST DAY!

I'd like to end this chapter with a brief pep talk about Feast Day – or maybe it's a pepperoni talk! Because on Feast Day you should have that pepperoni, and the pizza, and whatever other toppings, side dishes, beverages and snacks strike your fancy. Truly, on Feast Day there are no restrictions and no forbidden foods. There are no rules whatsoever, unless 'Enjoy yourself' is a rule!

Remember, the Every-Other-Day Diet works *because* you diet only every other day. The unrestricted day off from dieting gives your body the calories and nutrients it needs for a day of modified fasting. The modified fast creates a condition that helps you not overeat. Both days are necessary. Diet Day and Feast Day work *together* to produce sustained and safer weight loss.

If you're reading this book, it's likely that all the diets you've tried have failed. The Every-Other-Day Diet is unique – and uniquely effective. And Feast Day is the day of food and fun that makes it work!

---

### EOD – EASY AS 1-2-3!

**1.** On Feast Day, eat all the food you want, and eat any kind of food you want.

**2.** Don't worry about bingeing on Feast Day – you won't.

**3.** You're not changing *what* you eat – you're changing your *pattern* of eating.

---

## CHAPTER 4

# Every-Other-Day Dieting, Quick and Easy

*These lunch and dinner recipes are only 400 calories – but they taste like a million!*

If you like to prepare your own lunch or dinner on Diet Day, and you're someone who enjoys perusing and choosing recipes and making meals, you probably look for a couple of key features in those that you make on a regular basis. You want them to be:

- *simple* – with a limited number of easy-to-find ingredients (complex recipes are so annoying)
- *speedy* – you don't want to spend too much time in the kitchen, and if you're hungry, you want to eat soon

- *scrumptious* – why bother making food if it's not tasty
- *surprising* – variety is the spice of life (and of lunch and dinner . . . )
- *filling* – you want meals that satisfy your appetite, rather than leaving you hungry

Well, you're in luck – because all of these benefits are just what the recipes in the Every-Other-Day Diet deliver. And that's because our recipe developer, Stephanie Karpinske, MS, RD, is an old hand at creating delicious recipes for diets and diet books. So to fit the criteria above for the recipes in the Every-Other-Day Diet, she made sure that:

- no recipe has an ingredient list of more than seven items
- cooking and preparation times are always under 30 minutes, and frequently under 20, so you're out of the kitchen fast
- the food is consistently tasty (at least Bill and I and our respective spouses thought so when we tested the recipes – and we're pretty sure you'll agree)
- the food is fun, too – it's amazing how much freshness and originality Stephanie packed into these meals and snacks
- the recipes are filling too because they feature appetite-satisfying protein and fibre

We've provided 28 days' worth of 400-calorie lunches, 28 days of 400-calorie dinners and 28 days of 100-calorie snacks. As you learned in chapter 2, you'll eat *either* lunch *or* dinner on Diet Day – your choice. Add the snack when it feels best to you, perhaps at mid-morning, mid-afternoon or at bedtime.

Before you start cooking, here are some points to take into account as you look at the recipes.

***Relax – the Every-Other-Day Diet is Simple to Follow.*** While writing this chapter, we reviewed the introductions to the recipe sections of many other diet books – and were they ever complicated! There are endless lists of foods to eat and not to eat. There are 'steps', 'phases' and 'waves' – time periods when you're asked to switch from one set of foods and/ or recipes to another. And the recipes themselves often seem like they might challenge even the most experienced chef, with long lists of ingredients and lengthy preparation times. No wonder so many people don't stick with their diets!

But you'll find none of this in the recipes in this chapter. What you will find are easy preparation, good flavour and one simple dietary rule: stick to 500 calories on Diet Day.

***Make your own meal plan.*** Speaking of simplicity, we didn't create a Meal Plan out of these lunches, dinners and snacks. That's because we wanted to give you maximum flexibility in choosing what meal to eat on Diet Day.

Maybe you want to eat lunch on Monday, dinner on Wednesday, dinner on Friday and lunch on Sunday? Go right ahead! Plus, feel free to mix and match the 28 snacks, making all of them over two months of Diet Days or choosing a few you especially like to make over and over again. In other words, you won't need a personal assistant to follow the EOD Diet!

**Brands** – when a brand-name product is mentioned it's just an example, chosen because the calorie count of that particular product is lower than similar ones.

If you decide to use a different product, check the calorie count of the product in the recipe against that of the one you're substituting to ensure that it is the same in both.

Sometimes we mention just a type of product, such as a low-fat salad dressing, where several brands are at the same level in terms of calories – we would then specify the rough calorie count to guide you (see below).

**Salad dressings/ mayonnaise** – where light, reduced-calorie or reduced-fat dressings and mayonnaise are specified, aim for a brand containing around 10–20 calories per tablespoon (15 ml) for salad dressing and around 35–40 calories per tablespoon (15g) for mayonnaise. There are several brands and supermarket own-brand versions available.

**Salt** – feel free to add salt as you wish. Where salt is listed as an ingredient, we found the recipe tasted better with a dash of it, otherwise, follow your own preferences and enjoy!

**Cheese** – we have used full-fat cheese where it didn't exceed the calorie count because my research shows that people who eat high-fat foods actually lose *more* weight on the EOD Diet, as long as they don't eat too many calories. Where full-fat cheese did exceed the calorie count, however, the recipe includes the reduced-fat variety.

**Tips and health info** – at the end of many of the recipes you'll find either a tip to ease shopping or preparation, or 'Health Info' about a particular, good-for-you ingredient.

**Satisfaction: you'll find plenty!** It's amazing how much food (and good flavour) Stephanie has packed into these

400-calorie lunches and dinners and 100-calorie snacks. They're delicious, nutritious and fun to eat. They're also filling, with plenty of appetite-satisfying protein and fibre. Enjoy!

---

## USING READY MEALS ON DIET DAY

I know, I know: you're very busy, and you'd like to minimise time spent in the kitchen. Well, one way to cut cooking time on Diet Day is by using ready meals.

Many food manufacturers produce ready meals, and all the major supermarkets stock these frozen or chilled foods. Simply stroll to the refrigerator section, and you'll find not only traditional English dishes, but also Italian, Indian, Chinese, Mexican and Thai. The meals come in individual portions or multiple-portion packs. They're tasty, and only need minimal preparation before you can sit down and eat.

Some ready meals are high in calories. However, most now have clear front-of-pack labelling, usually as 'traffic lights' in the format recommended by the UK Food Standards Agency. These labels allow you to see at a glance the calorie content of the meal – whether it's low (green), medium (amber) or high (red) in calories.

Often, ready meals with the lowest calories are those in the 'healthy eating' ranges offered by stores. Many of them have around 400 calories per serving – perfect for Diet Day. But you don't need to limit your choices to just these ranges; by checking labels, you'll find other ready meals with around the same calorie content.

## TWO TIPS FOR USING READY MEALS

1. Keep it to 400 calories: look for meals providing around 400 calories per portion. Add a 100-calorie snack and you're set for Diet Day. Keep in mind, however, that some packages contain two or more servings, so check the label carefully for the per-serving level of calories.
2. Add some vegetables: if you'd like a low-calorie side dish, try a small bag of ready-washed salad, garnishing it with no-fat dressing. (A handful of salad greens is about 10 calories.) If the ready-made meal is 300 calories or so, consider adding a portion of easy-cook tinned or frozen vegetables, which weighs in at about 120 calories.

Here's a list of a few of the manufacturers and retailers that offer ready meals of around 400 calories per serving. Enjoy!

- Asda: Good For You! or Chosen by You: Reduced Calorie
- Birds Eye
- The City Kitchen
- The Co-op: Good Life
- Innocent
- Marks and Spencer: Count on Us or Fuller Longer
- Morrisons: NuMe
- Quorn
- Sainsbury's: Be Good to Yourself or Balanced or My Goodness

- Tesco: Light Choices or Eat Live Enjoy
- Waitrose: Love Life or You Count
- WeightWatchers
- Wiltshire Farm Foods

## 400-CALORIE LUNCHES

### *Italian Quinoa Salad*

40g dry quinoa
55g tuna in spring water or brine, drained
80g tinned chickpeas, rinsed and drained
½ small cucumber, peeled and chopped
5 Kalamata olives, stones removed and chopped
2 tablespoons light or low-fat Italian-style or vinaigrette
    dressing

Cook quinoa according to the instructions on the packet, then
leave to cool.

Place cooked quinoa in a medium bowl. Add remaining
ingredients and mix to combine. If desired, chill before serving.

**Health info:** Quinoa (pronounced *keen-wah*) is a gluten-free grain, with
none of the type of protein found in wheat and rye that many people
are trying to avoid for better health. Quinoa has a mild flavour that
mixes well with other ingredients, and it's rich in protein, making it a
great choice for vegetarians.

## Turkey and Avocado Sandwich

1 Warburtons Sandwich Thin
1 Laughing Cow Light cheese triangle
110g cold turkey breast, thinly sliced
2–3 tomato slices
⅕ of an avocado, peeled, stone removed and thinly sliced

Split Sandwich Thin open. Spread one half with the cheese triangle, then top with the turkey slices, tomato, avocado and remaining half of the Sandwich Thin.

Serve with: 1 piece of fresh fruit or a 20–25g bag of any flavour Pop-Chips or other reduced fat/light crisps (giving around 100 calories per bag).

**Health info:** Tomatoes are rich in lycopene, an anti-cancer compound. Eating avocado *with* tomatoes increases the body's absorption of lycopene by an amazing 200 to 400 per cent.[1]

## BBQ Chicken and Broccoli Wrap

80g roast chicken breast, finely sliced
55g tinned sweetcorn, drained
70g chopped broccoli
2 teaspoons barbecue sauce
1 tablespoon reduced-fat creamy or Ranch salad dressing
1 small (35–40g) tortilla wrap (100 per cent wholewheat, if
    available)

Place the chicken, sweetcorn, broccoli, barbecue sauce and salad dressing in a medium bowl. Mix until everything is coated. Place mixture on the tortilla wrap and carefully roll up. If desired, cut in half before serving.

**Preparation tip:** You could also use plain cooked chicken breast. It has fewer calories than roast chicken, but also less flavour.

## Tortellini Salad

½ small pack (125g) fresh filled tortellini (such as four cheese, spinach and ricotta or mushroom)

75g fresh mangetout

75g chopped yellow sweet pepper

75g chopped red sweet pepper

2 tablespoons low-fat/light sesame ginger salad dressing (or similar Asian-style dressing)

Cook, drain and cool the tortellini according to the instructions on the packet, then add the mangetout, peppers and dressing. Chill before serving, if desired.

**Shopping tip:** You'll find fresh filled tortellini in the chilled section of the supermarket.

## Kidney Bean and Corn Salad

190g tinned kidney beans, rinsed and drained

110g tinned sweetcorn, drained

150g chopped green pepper

1 small tomato, chopped

½ small avocado, peeled, stone removed and chopped

1 tablespoon red wine vinegar

¼ teaspoon cumin

Mix all the ingredients together in a medium bowl. If desired, season with salt.

**Health info:** Several studies from Arizona State University show that adding vinegar to a meal can help control post-meal spikes of blood sugar, probably because the acetic acid in the vinegar partially blocks an enzyme that breaks down carbohydrate.[2]

## Ham, Apple and Cheddar Sandwich

1 teaspoon light or reduced-fat butter
1 wholegrain muffin, toasted
110g lean ham, thinly sliced
1 small apple, thinly sliced
1 x 25g slice reduced-fat mature Cheddar cheese

Spread the butter on the bottom half of the muffin. Top
with the ham, then 3–4 slices apple, then the Cheddar cheese
and the muffin top. Serve the remaining apple slices with the
sandwich.

## Roast Beef Roll

50g bottled roasted red peppers in brine, drained and
    chopped
5 small Kalamata olives, stones removed and chopped
1 teaspoon red wine vinegar
100g lean roast beef, thinly sliced
1 x 25g slice reduced-fat Cheddar cheese
1 small (50g) wholegrain bread roll

Preheat oven to 350°F/180°C/gas mark 4.

Place red peppers, olives and vinegar in a small bowl. Mix to
combine, then set aside.

Place the roll on an oven-safe tray. Split the roll open and
top with the roast beef and cheese. Cook in the preheated oven
for 2–3 minutes or until the roll is toasted and the cheese has
melted. Remove from the oven and top with the pepper–olive
mixture.

## Chicken and Cashew Coleslaw

300g coleslaw mix (i.e. without mayonnaise) or 150g sliced
    white cabbage/100g grated carrot and 50g chopped
    onion, mixed

110g cooked chicken breast, chopped

75g fresh mangetout

2 tablespoons reduced fat/light vinaigrette or Asian-style
    dressing

10 dry-roasted cashews, chopped

Place everything except the cashews in a large bowl. Mix until
the vegetables are evenly coated with the dressing. Leave to rest
for 10 minutes to allow the dressing to soak into the coleslaw. Toss
in the cashews immediately before serving.

**Health info:** A study from the University of Montreal shows that cashew
extracts may be anti-diabetic, helping muscles to use blood sugar.[3]

## Taco Salad

1 small bag mixed salad leaves

25g reduced-fat Cheddar cheese, grated

110g cooked chicken breast, chopped

$1/2$ red sweet pepper, deseeded and chopped

1 tablespoon light or low-fat creamy or Ranch salad dressing

2 tablespoons bottled or fresh salsa

10 bite-sized tortilla chips, broken into pieces

Place salad leaves, cheese, chicken and pepper in a medium
bowl. In a separate smaller bowl, stir together the dressing and
salsa. Pour dressing over salad and toss to coat. Top with broken
tortilla chips before serving.

**Health info:** A bag of mixed salad greens delivers far more calcium,
vitamin C and vitamin A than the same amount of iceberg lettuce.

## Turkey and Hummus Wrap

1 tablespoon (25g) reduced-fat hummus (any flavour)
1 small (40g) tortilla wrap
80g (4 small thin slices) cold turkey breast
5–6 leaves fresh baby spinach
3–4 tomato slices

Spread the hummus on the tortilla wrap. Top with the turkey slices, spinach and tomato. Roll up and cut in half.

Serve with: 1 piece of fresh fruit or a 20–25g bag of any flavour Pop-Chips or other reduced fat/light crisps (giving approximately 100 calories per bag).

**Shopping and preparation tip:** The calories in reduced-fat hummus can vary by brand: choose a brand with approximately 50–55 calories per tablespoon (25g). If you go for a type with more calories (check the label), then adjust the amount used accordingly.

## Mango Chicken Salad

110g cooked chicken breast, sliced
2 tablespoons chopped celery
2 tablespoons chopped red onion
5 dry-roasted almonds, chopped
60g fat-free (0% fat) Greek yogurt
1 tablespoon mango chutney
30g (3 slices) Ryvita

Place the chicken, celery, red onion and almonds in a medium bowl. In a separate smaller bowl, mix together the yogurt and chutney. Pour over the chicken mixture and mix until combined. If desired, season with salt. Serve salad on or with Ryvita.

**Health info:** Studies show that almonds aid weight control and deliver several other health benefits, including satisfying the appetite, helping to control blood-sugar levels in healthy people and those with type-2 diabetes and lowering bad LDL cholesterol (see p. 30).[4]

## Tuna and White Bean Salad

30g uncooked mini shell pasta
110g tinned tuna in brine or spring water, drained
130g tinned cannellini or haricot beans, rinsed and drained
½ medium cucumber, peeled and chopped
35g reduced-fat feta cheese
2 tablespoons light Italian-style salad dressing

Cook the pasta according to instructions on the packet, then drain and leave to cool.

Place cooked pasta in a medium bowl. Add tuna, beans, cucumber, feta cheese and dressing. Toss to coat. Chill before serving, if desired.

**Shopping tip:** Tuna in brine or spring water has fewer calories per serving than tuna in oil.

## Turkey Couscous Salad

40g dry wholewheat couscous
85g cooked turkey breast, cubed
1 small orange, peeled, sectioned and cut into bite-sized pieces
1 tablespoon sultanas or dried cranberries
1 spring onion, chopped
2 tablespoons light salad dressing

Cook couscous according to the instructions on the packet, then leave to cool.

Place couscous in a medium bowl. Add turkey, orange pieces, dried fruit, spring onion and dressing. Toss to coat. Chill before serving, if desired.

**Preparation tip:** When making couscous, be sure to follow the cooking instructions on the packet closely. If you add too much water, you'll end up with soggy, rather than fluffy grain. And if you cook the couscous too long it can stick to the bottom of the pan.

## Turkey and Cranberry Bagel

1 WeightWatchers bagel
1 tablespoon cranberry sauce
75g smoked turkey breast, thinly sliced
1 thin slice (25g) reduced-fat mature Cheddar cheese
1 leaf romaine or cos lettuce

Split open the bagel. Spread cranberry sauce on the bottom half, then top with turkey, cheese, lettuce and bagel top. Cut in half to serve.

## Ham and Pear Wrap

1 tablespoon reduced-fat soft cheese spread
1 teaspoon Dijon mustard
1 multigrain medium (20cm) tortilla
110g lean ham, thinly sliced
1 thin slice red onion, separated into rings
1 medium pear

Mix the soft cheese and mustard together and spread on the tortilla. Top with the ham and red onion. Cut the pear into thin slices, placing a third of them on top of the red onion. Roll up the tortilla, then cut in half. Serve with the remaining pear slices.

**Health info:** Red onions are one of the richest sources of quercetin, a powerful antioxidant that studies have linked to lower blood pressure, lower LDL cholesterol (see p. 30), fewer allergy symptoms and less fatigue during exercise.[5]

### Chicken and Pasta Soup

110g cooked chicken breast, chopped
50g frozen mixed vegetables
750ml chicken stock
45g dried macaroni

Combine the chicken, vegetables and stock in a small saucepan and bring to the boil. Add the pasta, then simmer for 10–12 minutes or until the pasta and vegetables are tender.

### Ham and Butter Bean Soup

110g lean cooked ham, chopped
190g tinned butterbeans, rinsed and drained
$\frac{1}{2}$ small courgette, chopped
$\frac{1}{2}$ yellow pepper, deseeded and chopped
625ml chicken stock
$\frac{1}{8}$ teaspoon black pepper

Combine all the ingredients in a small saucepan. Bring to the boil, then simmer for 12–15 minutes or until vegetables are tender.

**Shopping tip:** There's a lot of variation in sodium (salt) levels in shop-bought chicken stock cubes. Look out for those labelled 'reduced salt'.

### Turkey and Orzo Soup

110g cooked turkey breast, chopped
70g chopped kale
70g chopped white button mushrooms
750ml chicken stock
45g dried orzo pasta
1 tablespoon grated Parmesan cheese

Combine turkey, kale, mushrooms and stock in a small saucepan. Bring to the boil, then add the orzo and simmer for 10–12 minutes or until the vegetables are the desired tenderness and the orzo is cooked. Top with Parmesan cheese before serving.

**Health info:** Kale boosts the body's level of nitric oxide, relaxing arteries and helping to control blood pressure.

### Edamame Pasta Salad

30g dried penne pasta
75g frozen shelled edamame (soybeans)
½ yellow pepper, deseeded and chopped
75g cherry or baby plum tomatoes, halved
2 tablespoons light balsamic salad dressing or light vinaigrette
2 tablespoons reduced-fat feta cheese

Cook the pasta and beans according to the instructions on the packet. Drain and leave to cool.

Place the pasta and beans in a medium bowl. Add remaining ingredients and toss to coat. Chill before serving, if desired.

**Health info:** Edamame (pronounced *ed-ah-ma-may*), also known as soybeans, are a standard appetiser in Japanese restaurants. They are rich in phytoestrogens, a plant-based, weaker version of oestrogen, and may help to ease the hot-flush symptoms of menopause. You can find frozen shelled soybeans in some larger supermarkets.

### Asian Chicken Salad

110g cooked chicken breast, chopped
80g pineapple chunks, drained
1 tablespoon chopped red pepper
5 almonds, chopped

100g microwavable brown rice (such as Uncle Ben's Express
Rice or Tilda Steamed Rice), cooked according to instructions on the packet
50g bagged salad leaves
2 tablespoons reduced-fat/light Asian-style salad dressing

Place all the ingredients in a medium bowl. Gently toss to
combine. Chill before serving, if desired.

**Health info:** Pineapple is rich in bromelain, an enzyme that aids
digestion and reduces inflammation.

## Ham and Rice Salad

75g frozen peas, defrosted
100g microwavable brown rice (such as Uncle Ben's Express
Rice or Tilda Steamed Rice), cooked according to instructions on the packet
75g lean cooked ham, chopped
1 plum tomato, chopped
80g chopped romaine or cos lettuce
2 tablespoons reduced-fat creamy or Ranch salad dressing

Place all ingredients in a medium bowl. Gently toss to combine.
Chill before serving, if desired.

**Health info:** Brown rice is a whole grain, and a study from Wake Forest
University shows that eating 2–3 servings of whole grains daily can
significantly lower your risk of heart disease.[6]

## Thai Noodle Salad

30g dried wholewheat spaghetti or noodles
½ red pepper, deseeded and chopped
75g cooked chicken breast, sliced or chopped
2 spring onions, chopped

2 tablespoons peanut satay stir-fry sauce
10 dry-roasted peanuts, whole or chopped

Cook spaghetti or noodles according to the instructions on the packet. Drain and leave to cool.

Place the spaghetti or noodles in a medium bowl. Add the pepper, chicken, spring onion, peanut sauce and peanuts. Gently toss to combine. Chill before serving, if desired.

**Health info:** Peanuts get bad press as potential allergens. But if you're not allergic to them, they're very good for you – research shows roasted peanuts eaten with a meal can help to control blood sugar.[7]

## Chicken and Bacon Lettuce Wraps

3 slices cooked lean back bacon
110g cooked chicken breast, sliced or chopped
75g diced fresh tomato
2 tablespoons reduced-fat creamy or Ranch salad dressing
2–3 large lettuce leaves

Place the bacon, chicken, tomato and dressing in a medium bowl. Mix to combine. Fill the lettuce leaves with the chicken mixture, then roll leaves up to serve.

Serve with: 1 small piece of fresh fruit.

## Corn and Bean Burrito

150g refried beans
2 tablespoons bottled or fresh salsa
1 multigrain medium (20cm) tortilla
40g tinned sweetcorn, drained
10g shredded lettuce
25g reduced-fat Cheddar cheese, grated

Place the beans in a covered microwave-safe dish and heat on high for 45 seconds–1 minute, stirring halfway through. If beans aren't heated through, return to the microwave for a few seconds more. Remove beans from the microwave and stir in the salsa. Spread the bean mixture over the tortilla, then top with sweetcorn, lettuce and cheese. Roll the ends of the tortilla towards the centre, then roll up from the side to serve.

## Loaded Baked Potato

1 medium baking potato
2 tablespoons low-fat onion and garlic or sour cream and chive dip
$1/4$ teaspoon black pepper
150g chopped frozen broccoli
75g lean cooked ham, chopped

Scrub the potato and prick the sides several times with a fork. Place in the microwave and cook on high for 5–6 minutes or until tender. Split open the top of the potato and scoop out two-thirds of the flesh into a small bowl. Add the dip and pepper, then mix to combine. Scoop the potato mixture back into the skin. Cook broccoli according to the instructions on the packet, and warm ham in the microwave, if desired. Top the potato with the broccoli and ham.

**Health info:** Potatoes are loaded with potassium – an important mineral for preventing and lowering high blood pressure.

## Spicy Beef Chilli

110g extra lean minced beef
240g tinned chopped tomatoes, undrained
170g tinned kidney beans, rinsed and drained

130g bottled or fresh chunky salsa
125ml water
$\frac{1}{2}$ teaspoon chilli seasoning or chilli powder
1 tablespoon grated reduced-fat Cheddar cheese

Brown the minced beef in a small to medium saucepan over medium-high heat until cooked through. Drain fat, if necessary. Add the chopped tomatoes, beans, salsa, water and chilli seasoning. Bring to the boil, then simmer for 10-15 minutes. Top with the grated cheese before serving.

**Health info:** Kidney beans deliver soluble fibre, which can help to control blood cholesterol and blood-sugar levels.

## Roast Beef with Cucumber Sauce

$\frac{1}{2}$ cucumber, peeled, deseeded and chopped
35g reduced-fat sour cream or crème fraîche
1 tablespoon chopped red onion
$\frac{1}{2}$ tablespoon chopped fresh dill
$\frac{1}{8}$ teaspoon salt
1 wholewheat pitta bread
110g lean cold roast beef, thinly sliced

Place the cucumber, sour cream, red onion, dill and salt in a small bowl. Mix well. Cut pitta in half and split open. Divide roast beef between pitta halves. Top with the cucumber sauce.

**Health info:** A study in *Stroke: Journal of the American Heart Association* links eating cucumber (and other fruits and vegetables with white flesh, like apples and pears) to a 52 per cent lower risk of stroke.[8]

### Mediterranean Tuna-topped Tomato

140g tinned tuna in brine or spring water, drained
½ tablespoon olive oil
5 small Kalamata olives, stones removed and chopped
1 tablespoon chopped red onion
35g reduced-fat feta cheese
1 medium tomato

Place the tuna, olive oil, olives, red onion and feta cheese in a small bowl. Gently mix to combine. Cut out the tomato stem, then slice tomato into quarters. Top with the tuna mixture.

## 400-CALORIE DINNERS

### Herby Crumble-crusted Cod

150g piece white fish such as cod, coley, hake, haddock, about 1¼cm thick
60g low-fat buttermilk
2 tablespoons cornmeal or breadcrumbs
½ teaspoon lemon-pepper seasoning (optional)
⅛ teaspoon dried dill or parsley

Preheat the oven to 425°F/220°C/gas mark 7.

Place the fish in a freezer bag. Pour the buttermilk into the bag and seal. Turn the bag from side to side to coat the cod, then set aside. Combine the breadcrumbs, pepper and herbs in a small bowl. Remove the fish from the bag and place it in the breadcrumb mixture. Turn to coat all sides of the fish. Place fish in a shallow baking dish that's been lightly coated with non-stick cooking spray. Lightly spray the top of the fish with the cooking spray. Bake in the preheated oven for 12–15 minutes, turning once. The fish is done when it flakes easily with a fork.

Serve with: 250g (prepared weight) packet mashed potato made up according to the instructions on the packet.

**Health info:** Even a little bit of parsley does the body good – research shows the herb may help fight heart disease, diabetes and cancer.

## Spaghetti and Meatballs

45g wholewheat dried spaghetti
4 fresh turkey or beef meatballs or 6 meat-free meatballs
125g tomato pasta sauce
$1/2$ teaspoon Italian seasoning or $1/4$ teaspoon each dried basil
    and dried oregano

Cook the pasta according to the instructions on the packet, then drain and set aside.

Cook the meatballs according to the instructions on the packet. Place tomato sauce and seasonings in a small saucepan and simmer until sauce is warmed. Add the meatballs to the sauce and stir to combine. Serve the meatballs and sauce over the cooked spaghetti. Serve with: 60g cooked green beans.

**Health info:** Oregano is another health-giving spice, with research linking it to the prevention of a wide range of diseases and conditions, including infections, pre-diabetes and high cholesterol.

## Pepperoni French Bread Pizza

$1/3$ small French baguette (50g)
60g tinned chopped tomatoes with herbs, drained
30g (6 small slices) pepperoni
4 white button mushrooms, thinly sliced
35g reduced-fat mozzarella cheese, grated
chopped fresh basil

Preheat the oven to 425°F/220°C/gas mark 7.

Slice the bread in half and place on a baking sheet. Top each half with the chopped tomatoes, spreading evenly to cover. Add the pepperoni slices, mushrooms and cheese. Bake in the preheated oven until the cheese has melted and is starting to brown. Remove from the oven and top with chopped basil.

Serve with: tossed salad made using 60g bagged salad leaves, 75g cherry or baby plum tomatoes and 2 tablespoons light salad dressing.

## Chicken Enchiladas

55g cold chicken breast, chopped
130g tinned beans (such as kidney or cannellini), rinsed and
    drained
65g spicy tomato pasta sauce
2 tablespoons grated reduced-fat Cheddar cheese
2 small corn tortillas (or 1 medium multigrain tortilla)

Preheat the oven to 400°F/200°C/gas mark 6.

Combine the chicken, beans, 2 tablespoons of the tomato sauce and 1 tablespoon of the cheese in a medium bowl. Place the mixture on the tortillas. Carefully roll up the tortillas and place in a small baking dish. (It's OK if the filling spills out the sides.) Spoon the remaining sauce over the top of the enchiladas, then top with the remaining cheese. Cook in the preheated oven for 10–12 minutes or until the filling is warmed.

## BBQ Pork Chops with Apple-topped Sweet Potato

$1/2$ teaspoon barbecue herb and spice blend

1 x (110g) lean, boneless pork chop, about $1^1/4$cm thick

1 medium (150g) sweet potato

100g apple sauce

$1/4$ teaspoon cinnamon

Rub the barbecue seasoning on both sides of the pork chop. Spray a medium frying pan with non-stick cooking spray. Place the pork chop in the pan and cook over medium–high heat for 4–5 minutes on each side or until it is cooked through. While the pork chop is cooking, scrub the sweet potato, then prick all around the outside of it with a fork. Microwave on high for 7–10 minutes or until tender. Split the top of the potato open. Mix the apple sauce with cinnamon, then top the sweet potato with the apple sauce. Serve with pork chop.

> **Health info:** Sweet potatoes are loaded with the antioxidant alpha-carotene, and a ten-year study from the Centers for Disease Control and Prevention showed that people with the highest blood levels of alpha-carotene had a 39 per cent lower risk of death during the study than those with low levels.[9]

## Steak and Peppers

1 x (110g) lean sirloin steak, about 2cm thick

2 garlic cloves

salt and pepper

$1/2$ tablespoon olive oil

$1/2$ green pepper, deseeded and thinly sliced

$1/2$ red pepper, deseeded and thinly sliced

$1/3$ small onion, thinly sliced

Preheat the grill.

Trim the steak of any visible fat, then place on the grill-pan tray. Cut one garlic clove in half and rub the cut sides on both sides of the steak. Sprinkle with salt and pepper. Grill 10cm from the heat for 8–12 minutes or until the steak is cooked as desired, turning once. Keep an eye on the steak while it grills, as it can burn quickly.

For the pepper mixture, heat the oil in a medium frying pan. Add the peppers and onion and sauté for a few minutes over medium–high heat. If the peppers start to burn, add water, a tablespoon at a time, as needed. Chop the remaining clove of garlic and add to the pan. Continue to sauté for a few minutes more, until the peppers and onion are just tender. Serve peppers and onion with the steak.

> **Preparation tip:** When you're cooking with very little or no fat, food sometimes sticks to the pan. If that happens, add a small amount of water to the pan, 1 tablespoon at a time. (Be careful: water can splatter when you add it to a hot pan.)

### Cheesy Burger

130g extra lean minced beef
25g reduced-fat mature Cheddar cheese, grated
1 tablespoon finely chopped onion
1/8 teaspoon salt
1/8 teaspoon pepper
1 small hamburger bread roll (50g)
*Optional toppings:* lettuce, tomato, ketchup, mustard, gherkin

Preheat the grill.

Place the beef, cheese, onion, salt and pepper in a small to medium bowl. Mix together and form into a patty. Put the burger on the rack of a grill pan. Grill 10cm from the heat for

10-13 minutes or until cooked as desired. Remove the burger from the grill and serve on the bun with any of the optional toppers.

> **Health info:** Black pepper is rich in piperine, which research shows may help to ease arthritis, lower blood pressure, and prevent heart disease and Alzheimer's.[10]

## *Chicken Parmesan*

1 x (110g) skinless, boneless chicken breast
2 teaspoons olive oil
2 tablespoons breadcrumbs (panko best, if available)
$\frac{1}{2}$ teaspoon Italian seasoning
1 tablespoon grated Parmesan cheese
65g tomato pasta sauce
25g mozzarella cheese, grated

Preheat the oven to 425°F/220°C/gas mark 7.

Place the chicken on a baking sheet. Rub the oil on both sides of the chicken. In a small shallow bowl, mix together the breadcrumbs, Italian seasoning, and Parmesan cheese. Place the chicken in the breadcrumb mixture and turn to coat, pressing breadcrumbs into the chicken so they stick, then return the chicken to the baking sheet. Cook in the preheated oven for 20-25 minutes or until chicken is cooked through, turning once. Remove from the oven and top with the pasta sauce and mozzarella cheese, then return to the oven for a few minutes more until the cheese has melted.

## BBQ Salmon with Mango Salsa

1 x (110g) skinless salmon fillet, about 1cm thick
2 tablespoons barbecue sauce
160g chopped fresh mango
2 tablespoons chopped red onion
½ small cucumber, peeled and chopped
1 tablespoon chopped fresh coriander
juice of ½ small lime

Preheat the grill.

Place the salmon on the grill-pan tray, and grill 10cm from the heat for 4 minutes. Remove from the grill, brush with the barbecue sauce and grill for a further 2 minutes. Remove the salmon from the grill again, flip on to the other side and brush with the sauce. Grill for a further 2 minutes or until the fish flakes easily with a fork.

To make the salsa, place the mango, red onion, cucumber, coriander and lime juice in a small to medium bowl. Mix to combine and serve with the salmon.

**Health info:** Salmon and other oily fish is loaded with omega-3, a fat that is good for nearly every part of your body, including your brain (where it brightens mood), arteries (keeping them flexible and free of plaque), joints (easing aches and pains) and eyes (helping to prevent cataracts and other age-related eye problems).[11]

## Chicken Stir-fry

110g raw chicken fillets, sliced into thin strips
150g frozen stir-fry vegetables
2 tablespoons stir-fry sauce
200g microwavable brown rice (such as Uncle Ben's Express
  Rice or Tilda Steamed Rice), cooked according to the
  instructions on the packet

Lightly coat a medium frying pan with non-stick cooking spray. Add the sliced chicken fillets and cook over medium–high heat for 4–5 minutes. Add the frozen vegetables and stir-fry sauce. Cook for 4–5 minutes more or until the chicken is cooked through and the vegetables cooked as desired. Serve over brown rice.

### Ravioli with Vegetables

1 courgette, chopped
150g cherry tomatoes, halved
80ml chicken stock
60g fresh baby spinach
1/2 small packet (125g) fresh filled ravioli, cooked according to the instructions
2 tablespoons grated Parmesan cheese

Spray a medium to large frying pan with non-stick cooking spray. Add the courgette and tomatoes and sauté over medium–high heat for 2–3 minutes. Add the stock and spinach and continue to sauté for 4–5 minutes or until the courgette is tender. Stir in the cooked ravioli just to combine. Remove from the heat and top with cheese before serving.

**Shopping and preparation tip:** You'll find a variety of fresh filled ravioli in the chilled section of the supermarket. Prepare it according to the instructions on the packet.

### Pasta with Cream Sauce

35g light/low-fat soft cheese
60ml skimmed milk
1/8 teaspoon salt
1 tablespoon grated Parmesan cheese
80g frozen peas, defrosted

150g (cooked weight) fresh pasta such as egg tagliatelle or
    spaghetti, cooked according to the instructions on the
    packet
coarse-ground black pepper

Whisk together the soft cheese, milk and salt in a small
saucepan. Bring to the boil, stirring constantly. Stir in the
Parmesan, then simmer over medium heat until the mixture starts
to bubble and thicken, stirring occasionally. Stir in the peas. Pour
the sauce over prepared pasta and toss until thoroughly coated.
Season with black pepper.

> **Shopping and preparation tip:** You'll find a variety of fresh pasta
> which work well in this dish, such as tagliatelle, spaghetti or linguine,
> in the chilled section of the supermarket. Prepare according to the
> instructions on the packet.

## Mini Meat Loaf with Mashed Potatoes

150g lean minced beef
1 teaspoon breadcrumbs
1 teaspoon dry French onion soup mix
2 teaspoons tomato ketchup

Preheat the oven to 450°F/230°C/gas mark 8.

Place the beef, breadcrumbs, onion soup mix and ketchup in a
small to medium bowl, and mix well to combine. Form the mixture
into a small oval-shaped loaf, and cook in the preheated oven
for 15–20 minutes or until cooked through. Keep an eye on the
meatloaf as it cooks as it can easily burn at this temperature.

Serve with: 250g (cooked weight) packet mashed potatoes,
prepared according to the instructions.

## Chicken Nachos

15g tortilla chips
50g cooked chicken, sliced or chopped
100g tinned beans (such as kidney, black-eyed or cannellini),
    rinsed and drained
50g reduced-fat mature Cheddar cheese, grated
1 large tomato, diced or 2 tablespoons bottled or fresh salsa
5 slices bottled jalapeño peppers (optional)

Preheat the oven to 375°F/190°C/gas mark 5.

Spread the tortilla chips out on a baking tray, so that they're touching but not piled on top of each other. Top the chips evenly with chicken, beans and cheese, then cook in the preheated oven for 5–8 minutes or until the cheese has melted. Remove from the oven and top with diced tomato and jalapeños, if using.

**Health info:** Jalapeños are rich in capsaicin, a compound that studies show helps to control appetite.[12]

## Sautéed Prawns with Kale and Pine Nuts

2 teaspoons olive oil
110g raw peeled prawns
1 garlic clove, thinly sliced
70g chopped kale
130g tinned cannellini or haricot beans, rinsed and drained
1 tablespoon pine nuts

Heat the oil in a medium frying pan. Add the prawns and sauté over medium–high heat for 2–3 minutes. Add the garlic and kale and sauté for a further 4–5 minutes or until the prawns are cooked and opaque. Stir in the beans. Remove from the heat and sprinkle with pine nuts before serving.

## Chicken with Spinach and Tomatoes

1 x (140g) skinless, boneless chicken breast
1 tablespoon olive oil
90g fresh baby spinach
1 garlic clove, thinly sliced
110g cherry tomatoes
80ml chicken stock
6 Kalamata olives, stones removed and sliced

Cut the chicken into medium strips. Heat the oil in a medium to large frying pan, add the chicken and sauté over medium-high heat for 3-4 minutes. Add the spinach, garlic and tomatoes and sauté for a further 2-3 minutes. Add the stock and sliced olives and simmer for 5-8 minutes, stirring occasionally, until the chicken is cooked through and the tomatoes are tender.

**Health info:** Garlic is *great* for you. When scientists from the UK reviewed all the scientific literature on garlic and health, they concluded that regular intake could help to prevent many age-related diseases, including heart disease, stroke and some types of cancer.

## Scallops with Pineapple Salsa

140g fresh or frozen scallops
½ teaspoon Cajun seasoning or Cajun herb and spice blend
2 teaspoons olive oil
240g fresh chopped pineapple
2 tablespoons chopped red onion
½ small green chilli pepper, deseeded and chopped
7 almonds, coarsely chopped

Defrost the scallops, if frozen, then rinse and pat dry with kitchen paper. Place in a medium bowl with the Cajun seasoning and toss until lightly coated. Heat the oil in a medium frying pan, add the scallops and cook over medium-high heat for 4–5 minutes or until scallops are opaque. Remove from the heat.

To make the salsa, place the pineapple, red onion, chilli pepper and almonds in a medium bowl and toss to combine. Serve with the scallops.

**Health info:** Enjoy that olive oil! A study on the Mediterranean diet in the *New England Journal of Medicine* shows that the diet can reduce heart attacks and stroke by 30 per cent compared to a low-fat diet, and that olive oil is probably the diet's most heart-healthy ingredient.

## Penne Primavera

60g dried penne pasta
1 tablespoon olive oil
½ small courgette, cut into thin strips
1 yellow or orange pepper, deseeded and cut into thin strips
70g sliced portobello or white button mushrooms
80ml chicken stock

Cook the pasta according to the instructions on the packet, then drain and set aside.

Heat the oil in a medium to large frying pan. Add the courgettes, pepper and mushrooms and sauté over medium-high heat for 5–6 minutes. Add the stock and continue to sauté for a few minutes more or until the vegetables are tender. Stir in the cooked pasta before serving.

**Shopping tip:** When buying pasta, try one of the many wholewheat blends now available. They have more nutrients and fibre than white pasta, yet taste almost the same.

## Egg and Cheese Casserole

2 large eggs
120ml skimmed milk
1/4 teaspoon wholegrain mustard
1/4 teaspoon black pepper
1 slice wholemeal bread, torn into bite-sized pieces
1 slice cooked back bacon, chopped
25g Cheddar cheese, grated

Preheat the oven to 400°F/200°C/gas mark 6.

Crack the eggs into a small bowl. Add the milk, mustard and pepper and whisk until combined. Set aside.

In an individual-sized casserole dish, place the bread, bacon and three-quarters of the cheese. Toss lightly to combine. Pour the egg mixture on top, then bake in the preheated oven for 20 minutes. Remove from the oven and top with the remaining cheese, then bake for a further 5–10 minutes or until a knife inserted in the centre comes out clean.

**Health info:** Don't be afraid of eggs, bacon and cheese on Diet Day. Studies show that a hearty dose of fat and protein helps you to feel full for hours, reducing hunger.[13] And my research shows you can eat *anything* on Diet Day and still improve risk factors for heart disease.

## Sirloin Steak with Mushroom Sauce

1/4 teaspoon black pepper
1/8 teaspoon garlic salt
1 x (110g) sirloin steak, about 2cm thick
70g sliced portobello mushrooms
70g sliced white button mushrooms
80g white lasagne sauce
1 spring onion, chopped (optional)

Preheat the grill.

Combine the pepper and garlic salt in a small bowl, then rub over both sides of the steak. Place the steak on the rack of a grill pan and grill 7.5cm from the heat for 8–12 minutes or until it is cooked as desired, turning once.

While the steak is cooking, prepare the mushroom sauce. Spray a medium frying pan with non-stick cooking spray. Add the mushrooms and sauté over medium–high heat for 5–7 minutes, adding water, 1 tablespoon at a time, if needed, to keep the mushrooms from burning. Stir in the white sauce and cook for a further 3–4 minutes or until the sauce is heated through. Pour over the steak and top with chopped spring onion, if using.

**Health info:** White button mushrooms strengthen the immune system, report scientists at Tufts University in the *British Journal of Nutrition*.[14]

## *Chicken Cacciatore*

40g dried fusilli pasta
1 x (110g) skinless, boneless chicken breast
½ green pepper, deseeded and chopped
70g sliced white button mushrooms
240g tinned chopped tomatoes with garlic and/or herbs, undrained

Cook the pasta according to the instructions on the packet, then drain and set aside.

Cut the chicken breast into bite-sized pieces. Spray a medium frying pan with non-stick cooking spray, add the chicken and cook over medium–high heat for 2–3 minutes, just to brown the outside of the chicken. Add the green pepper and mushrooms and sauté for a further 4–5 minutes or until the peppers are tender. Add the chopped tomatoes, reduce the heat and simmer for about 5 minutes more. Stir in the cooked pasta before serving.

## BBQ, Bacon and Pineapple Pizza

1 mini pizza base (75g)
1 tablespoon barbecue sauce
2 slices cooked lean back bacon
1 tablespoon chopped red onion
50g tinned pineapple pieces, drained
30g reduced-fat Cheddar or low-fat mozzarella, grated

Preheat the oven to 425°F/220°C/gas mark 7.

Place the pizza base on a baking sheet. Spread the barbecue sauce on top, then add the bacon, red onion and pineapple. Sprinkle the cheese on top and bake in the preheated oven for 10–12 minutes or until the cheese is bubbling and lightly browned.

## Rigatoni in Tomato Cream Sauce

60g dried rigatoni pasta
200g bottled or fresh tomato pasta sauce
80ml skimmed milk
¼ teaspoon Italian seasoning
2 tablespoons grated Parmesan cheese

Cook the pasta according to the instructions on the packet. Place the pasta sauce and milk in a small saucepan, bring to the boil, then reduce the heat and stir in the cheese. Simmer uncovered for 10–12 minutes or until the sauce thickens, stirring occasionally. Stir in the cooked pasta.

## Chicken and Bean Quesadillas

2 small flour tortillas (fajita-sized – around 30–35g each)
60g tinned refried beans
50g cooked skinless chicken breast, sliced or chopped
2 tablespoons reduced-fat Cheddar, grated
⅕ of a ripe avocado, peeled, stone removed and mashed

Spray a medium frying pan with non-stick cooking spray. Place one tortilla in the pan and spread refried beans on it, then top with the chicken and cheese. Place the other tortilla on a plate and spread one side with the mashed avocado. Place the avocado side of the tortilla on top of the one in the pan and press lightly so the quesadilla will hold together when you toss it. Spray the top of the quesadilla with non-stick cooking spray and cook over medium–high heat for 4–5 minutes on each side or until the cheese has melted and tortillas are lightly browned.

**Health info:** Avocados are among the best sources of monounsaturated fat, which studies show can help you control weight, lower bad LDL cholesterol (see p. 30) and balance blood sugar.

## Pork Chop with Sautéed Apples and Onions

1 teaspoon olive oil
1 x (140g) lean boneless pork chop, about 1¼cm thick
⅓ small onion, thinly sliced
1 small apple, cored and thinly sliced
125ml chicken stock
1 tablespoon balsamic vinegar

Heat the oil in a medium to large frying pan. Add the pork chop and cook over medium–high heat for 4–5 minutes on each side or until cooked through. Transfer the chop to a plate and cover to keep warm.

Place the onion and apple in the pan and sauté for 1-2 minutes to lightly brown the outsides. Pour in the stock and balsamic vinegar, bring to the boil, then simmer for 8-10 minutes or until the onion and apple are tender. (If the apple and onion mixture sticks to the pan, add a small amount of water.) Serve the apple mixture with the pork chop.

**Health info:** An apple a day might keep the cardiologist away. Researchers from Ohio State University found that people eating an apple a day for just one month had a 'tremendous' 40 per cent decrease in oxidised LDL cholesterol (see p. 30), the type that does the most damage to arteries.[15]

### Steak Tacos

1 x (110g) lean sirloin steak
120g tinned chopped tomatoes with chilli
2 small corn taco shells, such as Old El Paso
20g shredded lettuce
2 tablespoons reduced-fat grated Cheddar cheese

Cut the steak into thin strips. Spray a medium frying pan with non-stick cooking spray. Place the steak strips in the pan and sauté for 5-6 minutes over medium–high heat. Add the chopped tomatoes and cook for a further 5-6 minutes or until most of the liquid has evaporated. Divide the beef–tomato mixture between the two taco shells and top with the shredded lettuce and cheese.

### Chicken with Roasted Dijon Potatoes

100g diced red potatoes
2 teaspoons olive oil
1 teaspoon Dijon mustard
$1/8$ teaspoon salt

1 x (140g) chicken breast
1 tablespoon marinade, such as lemon and herb or honey and
    mustard

Preheat the oven to 425°F/220°C/gas mark 7.

Place red potatoes, oil, mustard and salt in a small bowl. Mix to coat, then transfer to a shallow oven-proof dish.

Place the chicken in an oven-proof baking dish, then pour marinade over it, turning to coat. Place the chicken and potatoes in the preheated oven and cook for 20-25 minutes or until the potatoes are tender and the chicken is cooked through (internal temperature of 170°F/80°C). If the chicken is done before the potatoes, remove it from the oven and cover to keep warm. Serve the chicken with the potatoes.

**Preparation tip:** Many marinades contain sugar and any remnants that run off the chicken tend to stick to the pan. So when preparing the chicken, line the baking pan with foil, which will make cleaning up quick and easy.

## Spicy Sausage and Rice

2 reduced-fat/healthy choice sausages, around 60-70 calo-
    ries each (such as WeightWatchers or Quorn)
80g tinned sweetcorn, drained
130g tinned kidney beans, rinsed and drained
100g microwavable brown rice (such as Uncle Ben's Express or
    Tilda Steamed Rice), cooked according to the instructions
    on the packet
2 tablespoons bottled or fresh salsa

Follow the instructions on the packet for cooking the sausages.

In a small microwave-safe bowl, combine the sweetcorn, beans, cooked rice and salsa. Microwave on high for 1 minute. Remove from the microwave and stir. If needed, microwave for another

30 seconds–1 minute or until the mixture is warmed. Slice the prepared sausages and serve with the rice.

**Shopping and preparation tips:** Rinsing tinned beans before using removes a lot of the salt: place them in a colander, rinse well with cold water, then let them sit for a minute to drain.

## 100-CALORIE SNACKS

### *Hummus Cucumber Boats*

1 medium cucumber
1½ tablespoons (35g) reduced-fat hummus (any flavour)
paprika or salt (optional)

Halve the cucumber lengthways. Use a spoon to hollow out the centre of each cucumber half, removing the seeds. Spread hummus in each cucumber half and sprinkle with paprika and/or salt, if using.

### *Frozen Berry Lolly*

90g 0% fat Greek yogurt
60ml orange juice
40g blueberries (fresh or frozen)
40g strawberries (fresh or frozen)

Place yogurt, juice and fruit in a blender or small food-processor and blend or process until smooth. Pour the mixture into a small plastic cup or ice-lolly mould. Place a lolly stick in the middle of the cup or lolly mould and freeze until solid. Remove from the cup or mould and serve.

**Health info:** Berries are superfruits. New studies show that regularly eating blueberries or strawberries can help to strengthen the immune system, lower blood pressure, balance blood sugar, improve memory and even help prevent precancerous lesions from turning into cancer.

## Fruit with Cheese Spread

1 Laughing Cow Light Blue Cheese Spread Triangle
½ small apple, sliced
½ small pear, sliced

Spread blue cheese on to apple and pear slices.

## PB&B Square

1 teaspoon reduced-fat peanut butter
1 plain digestive biscuit
¼ small (15cm) banana, sliced

Spread the peanut butter on to the digestive biscuit, then top with sliced banana.

**Health info:** Worried that eating a banana might spike your blood sugar? Relax. A study in the *International Journal of Food Sciences and Nutrition* shows that a banana is a healthy snack for anybody trying to regulate glucose levels, including people with diabetes.[16]

## Greek Yogurt Parfait

100g 0% fat Greek yogurt
2 strawberries, hulled and sliced
10g Kellogg's Froot Loops cereal

Place the yogurt in an ice-cream sundae glass, then top with the sliced strawberries and cereal.

### Carrot Sticks

2 x 25g slices cold turkey
1 teaspoon Dijon mustard
90g carrot sticks

Place the turkey slices on a plate and spread with the Dijon mustard. Cut the turkey into enough strips to allow one per carrot stick. Wrap the mustard side of each turkey strip around a carrot stick.

### Chocolate Stack

10g reduced-fat peanut butter
10g dark chocolate
4 strawberries, hulled

Spread the peanut butter over the chocolate. Slice one of the strawberries and place the slices on top of the chocolate. Serve with the remaining whole strawberries.

**Health info:** Dark chocolate is loaded with antioxidants that protect your arteries. Research shows that regularly eating a small amount of dark chocolate can help to lower blood pressure, LDL cholesterol (see p. 30) and the risk of heart disease and stroke.[17]

### Trail Mix Cereal

4 tablespoons Cheerios cereal
10 raisins

Mix the cereal and raisins together in a small bowl.

**Health info:** Canadian researchers have found that people who eat raisins as a snack feel fuller and eat fewer calories afterwards than those who choose grapes, crisps or biscuits.[18]

### Garden Fresh Toast

½ Warburtons Sandwich Thin
30g reduced-fat red pepper hummus
½ small cucumber, sliced
salt (optional)

Toast the Sandwich Thin, then spread with the hummus and top with sliced cucumbers. Lightly sprinkle with salt, if using.

### Tomatoes, Peppers and Cheese

½ medium tomato
½ yellow pepper, deseeded
30g mozzarella

Coarsely chop the tomato and pepper and place in a small bowl. Cut the cheese into small pieces and add to the bowl. Toss to combine.

### Apple Dippers

1 medium-sized eating apple
35g low-fat soft cheese spread
pinch of cinnamon

Core and slice the apple in quarters. Mix the soft cheese with the cinnamon. Eat the cheese, using apple quarters to dip.

### Fruity Crumpet Sticks

1 small (35g) crumpet, toasted
2 teaspoons light/reduced-fat soft cheese
1 teaspoon sugar-free fruit spread (any flavour)

Toast the crumpet, then spread with the cream cheese and then the fruit spread. Cut into 3–4 'sticks' to eat.

### *Tuna Salad Snack*

1 small tomato
60g tuna in brine or spring water, drained
1 tablespoon light creamy salad dressing

Cut out the tomato stem, then cut tomato into four wedges, leaving them connected at the bottom of the tomato. Place the tuna in a small bowl, add the dressing and mix to combine. Spoon the tuna over the cut tomato.

### *Chocolate Yogurt Sundae*

100g 0% fat Greek yogurt
10g Chocolate Cheerios cereal

Place the yogurt in a small bowl and top with the cereal.

### *Berry Bagel*

80g ripe strawberries, sliced
1 teaspoon sugar
½ WeightWatchers original bagel

Place the strawberries and sugar in a small bowl. Use the back of a fork to lightly mash the strawberries, taking care not to mash so much that they turn to liquid. You want them to be like a spreadable jam.

Toast the bagel, then top with the strawberry mixture.

## Tomato-basil Melt

½ wholegrain English muffin
1 small tomato, sliced
2–3 fresh basil leaves
15g reduced-fat/light mozzarella cheese, shredded

Preheat the grill.
Toast the English muffin half, then top with the tomato slices, basil and mozzarella cheese. Grill until the cheese has melted.

**Health info:** Two compounds in basil – orientin and vicenin – are potent inhibitors of free radicals, the errant, cell-damaging molecules that are a primary cause of ageing and chronic disease.

## Cinnamon Bagel with Orange Spread

½ WeightWatchers Bagel
15g reduced-fat/light soft cheese
2 teaspoons orange juice
½ teaspoon grated orange zest

Toast the half a bagel.
Place the soft cheese in a small bowl, add the orange juice and zest and mix well. Spread the cheese and orange mixture over the toasted bagel half.

**Health info:** Studies in *Nutrition Research*[19] and the *American Journal of Clinical Nutrition*[20] show that orange juice can lower bad LDL cholesterol and raise good HDL (see p. 30).

## Open-faced Cucumber Sandwich

½ Warburtons Sandwich Thin
50g low-fat cottage cheese
¼ cucumber, peeled and thinly sliced
dash pepper or salt

Toast the Sandwich Thin, then top with the cottage cheese and
cucumber slices. Sprinkle with pepper or salt.

**Health info:** A five-year study in *Nutrition* links regular intake of cottage
cheese and other calcium-rich dairy products with balanced blood
sugar and lower blood pressure, as well as less weight gain and a
smaller waistline.

## Strawberries and Cream Toast

½ Warburtons Sandwich Thin
1 Laughing Cow original cheese spread triangle
1 strawberry, sliced

Toast the Sandwich Thin, spread the cheese on top, then top
with strawberry slices.

## Almond-cherry Smoothie

250ml almond milk, such as Alpro
80g frozen dark sweet cherries
A handful of ice

Place almond milk, cherries and ice in a blender. Blend until
combined.

**Health info:** Health is a bowl of cherries. Studies at Boston University
School of Medicine show that cherries can help prevent gout (an
increasingly common health problem) or prevent gout attacks if you
already have the disease.[21] Other research shows that cherries lower

triglycerides and C-reactive protein, two risk factors for heart disease.[22] Cherries before bedtime can also improve sleep![23]

## Ham and Cheese Spirals

$1/2$ teaspoon mustard
1 x 30g slice lean, cold ham
1 large leaf lettuce
35g mozzarella cheese

Spread the mustard over the ham and place the lettuce on top. Cut the cheese into a stick shape and place in the centre of the lettuce. Roll up from one side to the other, then cut the roll-up into 2–3 pieces to serve.

**Health info:** A little mustard goes a long way – to better health. The mustard plant is in the cancer-fighting crucifer family, which includes broccoli, Brussels sprouts, kale and cabbage, and the mustard seed contains concentrated amounts of the same anti-cancer compounds found in those greens.

## Cinnamon Tortilla Strips

1 mini (fajita-sized) tortilla wrap, such as Mission Deli Mini Wraps
$1/2$ teaspoon sugar mixed with a pinch of cinnamon

Preheat the oven to 350°F/180°C/gas mark 4.

Place the tortilla on a cutting board. Spray one side with non-stick cooking spray and sprinkle cinnamon sugar evenly over the tortilla. Cut into 4–5 strips. Transfer strips to a baking sheet and place in the preheated oven for 6–9 minutes or until the strips are crisp and lightly browned.

## Creamy Dip with Peppers

60g WeightWatchers reduced-fat crème fraîche
1 tablespoon bottled or fresh chunky salsa
1 green pepper, deseeded and cut into thin strips

Place the crème fraîche and salsa in a small bowl and mix to combine. Serve with the green pepper strips.

## Crackers with Soft Cheese and Grated Carrot

25g Philadelphia Light soft cheese spread (any savoury flavour, such as garlic and herb/chive)
2 dark rye crispbreads
1 tablespoon grated carrot

Spread half of the soft cheese on each crispbread. Top each with ½ tablespoon shredded carrot.

**Health info:** Finnish scientists call it the 'Rye Factor' – the fact that blood-sugar levels stay uniquely balanced after a meal that includes rye bread.[24]

## Bananas with Crunchy Berry Topping

½ banana
1 tablespoon 0% fat Greek yogurt
10g (2 tablespoons) Kellogg's Special K Red Berries cereal

Cut the banana in half lengthways and place on a plate, cut-side up. Spread half of the yogurt on the cut surface of each banana slice. Top each with 1 tablespoon of the cereal.

### Berries with Fruit Dip

3 tablespoons plain 0% fat Greek yogurt

1½ teaspoons reduced-sugar jam or pure fruit spread (any flavour)

6 medium strawberries, hulled

Place the yogurt and jam or fruit spread in a small bowl. Mix to combine, then use as a dip for the strawberries.

**Health info:** Adding strawberries to the diet for eight weeks decreases total and LDL cholesterol (see p. 30), report scientists from Oklahoma State University in *Nutrition Research*.[25]

### Turkey-lettuce Rolls

75g sliced cold turkey breast

3 gherkin spears

3 small lettuce leaves

Wrap each slice of turkey around a gherkin spear, then wrap the lettuce around the turkey.

### Sweet and Salty Snack Mix

15g homemade or shop-bought air-popped popcorn (lightly salted)

2 tablespoons Chocolate Cheerios

Place the popcorn and cereal in a medium bowl and toss to combine.

**Health info:** Popcorn is a wholegrain and as a snack satisfies hunger and decreases appetite far better than crisps, according to a study in *Nutrition Journal*.[26]

## CHAPTER 5

# Every-Other-Day Dieting and Exercise

*A powerful combo for faster weight loss, a leaner body and a stronger heart*

The Every-Other-Day Diet is strong medicine. It helps you shed pounds, a must for better health if you're overweight or obese. It can lower several risk factors for heart disease, including total and LDL cholesterol, triglycerides and high blood pressure. It can balance blood sugar, helping prevent pre-diabetes and type-2 diabetes. And people on the diet report a range of other health benefits, like more energy, clearer thinking and fewer aches and pains.

But, as you'll read in this chapter, if you go on the EOD Diet *and* exercise, the strong medicine becomes stronger. Exercise is a uniquely powerful way to prevent disease and improve health. Among its many proven benefits, regular exercise can help you:

- build muscle, shed fat and control weight
- boost energy and banish fatigue
- brighten mood
- clear up depression and anxiety
- solve insomnia and other sleep problems
- ease the impact of chronic stress
- power up memory, concentration and learning ability
- prevent Alzheimer's disease
- balance blood sugar, preventing or reversing pre-diabetes and type-2 diabetes
- lower high blood pressure, a risk factor for heart attack and stroke
- increase good (HDL) cholesterol, protecting your arteries
- recover from a heart attack and prevent a second one
- prevent cancer and its recurrence
- prevent osteoporosis
- prevent osteoarthritis and relieve knee or hip pain from osteoarthritis
- prevent and relieve back pain

Research also shows that exercise can help reduce the burden of a wide range of other diseases and health problems, like addiction, chronic fatigue syndrome, chronic heart failure, COPD (chronic obstructive pulmonary disease), fibromyalgia, intermittent claudication (leg cramps and pain from poor circulation), irregular heartbeat (atrial fibrillation), menopausal problems, multiple sclerosis, neck and shoulder pain, Parkinson's disease, prostate problems and schizophrenia. And that list is far from complete.

*Bottom line:* exercise itself is powerful medicine for your body and mind. Combine it with the Every-Other-Day Diet, and you have an extra-strength approach to better health.

## EOD Dieting and Exercise: Better Together

As a scientist devoted to dealing with the twin epidemics of obesity and heart disease, I'm well aware of the health-enhancing powers of exercise, so I decided to conduct studies to see what would happen when people went on the Every-Other-Day Diet and exercised a couple of days per week.[1]

I'd already discovered that EOD dieters *could* exercise, a scientific finding that really surprised me; I thought that they would feel tired on Diet Day and avoid physical activity and exercise. But in a study of 16 people, published in *Nutrition Journal* in 2010, I found that people didn't slow down on Diet Day. And once I discovered that, I conducted another study on EOD dieting and exercise, trying to answer the following questions:

- Would a combination of the Every-Other-Day Diet and exercise trigger even more weight loss than EOD dieting alone?
- Would exercise make the EOD Diet even healthier for your heart?

- When was the best time of day to exercise on Diet Day, for maximum energy and minimum hunger? I didn't want people to be so hungry after exercising on Diet Day that they'd cheat on the diet.

The study involved 64 obese people (who were 2 stone 2lb (13.6kg) or more overweight) and lasted eight weeks. The participants were divided into four groups:

- *People doing EOD dieting and exercise.* For their exercise, the study participants worked out on either an exercise bike or an elliptical machine, which combines leg and arm movements. They started with workouts of 25 minutes, building up to 40 minutes by the end of the study. They also gradually increased exercise intensity, which we measured using a heart-rate monitor.
- *People doing only EOD dieting.*
- *People doing only exercise.*
- *People doing neither dieting nor exercise* (the control group).

My findings were remarkable: **people doing diet and exercise had twice as much weight loss as people doing only EOD dieting and not exercising.** Those who just dieted lost an average of 6.6lb (3kg) over the eight weeks of the study. But those who dieted and exercised lost *twice* as much weight, an average of 13.2lb (6kg). The people who exercised without dieting lost 2.2lb (1kg). The control group didn't lose any weight. An important point to note about the exercise-only group: it's *very* difficult to lose weight with exercise alone. Just do the maths. Starting today, you can reduce your food intake by 1000 calories and shed weight as your body burns stored fat for energy. But it would take several hours of walking to burn those same 1000 calories!

Exercise is a powerful *addition* to EOD dieting, as you're learning in this chapter. And if you exercise while on the EOD Diet, you're also much more likely to *maintain* weight loss, for reasons we'll explain – and permanent weight loss is the best result of any diet.

***Diet and exercise resulted in participants having more calorie-burning muscle.*** When most dieters lose weight, they lose body fat *and* muscle: 75 per cent fat and 25 per cent muscle. That's unfortunate, because losing muscle during dieting is a set-up for weight *regain*. Here's what happens: muscle is metabolically active – pound for pound, it burns *seven times* more calories than fat. So when a dieter has lost muscle during her diet, she burns fewer calories per day after the diet and slowly but surely gains back the weight she lost. That's the sad fate of nine out of ten dieters.

However, the group combining EOD dieting and exercise didn't lose *any* muscle during the eight weeks of the study – they lost only fat!

As I said a moment ago, that is a remarkable result, and it's probably one of the key factors that explains a major scientific finding I report at length in chapter 6, 'The Every-Other-Day Success Programme': EOD dieters *don't* regain their weight, compared to conventional dieters. Yes, the Every-Other-Day Diet is the first and only diet scientifically shown to help you not only lose weight – but also keep it off. You read that claim all the time, of course. But it's usually hope and hype. With the EOD Diet, it's *true*.

**People who dieted and exercised banished more tummy fat.** People who were exercising and dieting lost an average of 3" (7.6cm) from their waistlines. Those on the EOD Diet alone lost 2" (5cm). The exercisers who did not diet lost 1.2" (3cm).

**The EOD Diet + exercise group had higher HDL levels.** The EOD Diet + exercise group had the healthiest hearts, too. The exercise-and-diet combination produced a robust 12 per cent drop in bad, artery-clogging LDL – and a whopping 18 per cent increase in good, artery-clearing HDL. That's a very unique benefit. EOD dieting can lower LDL, and exercise can boost HDL, but only *combining them* does both.

**Summing up:** the combination of the Every-Other-Day Diet and exercise 'produces superior changes in body weight, body composition and lipid [fat] indicators of heart disease risk', when compared with EOD dieting or exercise alone, I wrote in the journal *Obesity* in 2013. Or, in non-scientific terms: if you want the best results, go on the Every-Other-Day Diet *and* exercise.

---

### STEVE'S STORY: 'I DON'T STOP EXERCISING ON DIET DAY'

*Weight loss: 1 stone 8lb (10kg)*

'I run for two miles, a couple of days a week,' says Steve, a 39-year-old sales director for a wireless phone company in Chicago, Illinois, and a former college football player who had seen his post-graduate weight creep up slowly, from 13 stone 3lb (83.9kg) to 16 stone 4lb (103.4kg).

On the Every-Other-Day Diet *and* exercise, he lost 1 stone 8lb (10kg) in 12 weeks, and he is looking forward to losing a lot more.

'I've always been a fairly active fellow,' he told us. 'But now that I've lost all that weight, I have more energy, my back and ankles don't hurt when I run and my cholesterol, blood pressure and blood-sugar levels are down.

'I don't stop exercising on Diet Day,' he continued. 'I run in the morning, drink a lot of water and I'm fine until lunch. I don't feel any ill effects whatsoever.'

---

The study described above showed what's happening to people's *bodies* on the EOD Diet. But what was happening in the *gym*? How did it feel to exercise on Diet Day? Did 500 calories fuel and support a workout, or were the EOD dieters weary, hungry and unhappy? My study answered those questions, too.

**It was easy to exercise on Diet Day.** The people in the study chose which day they'd exercise – Diet Day or Feast Day – and they chose both. In other words, people didn't have any problem exercising on Diet Day.

**People didn't overeat when they exercised.** When the participants in the study exercised in the *morning* on Diet Day, they were usually fine. They had a small snack mid-morning, ate lunch and didn't feel out of sorts; they cheated on the diet only about 10 per cent of the time. (Well, nobody's perfect.)

**There are three best times to exercise on Diet Day.**

Exercising in the afternoon wasn't the best strategy. Some participants reported being really hungry about 40 minutes after exercising if they exercised in the afternoon, and they cheated on the diet about 17 per cent of the time, often eating both lunch *and* dinner and exceeding their 500 calories. Cheating 17 per cent of the time isn't all that bad, in terms of sticking with the EOD Diet and losing weight. But it's not ideal. From that finding, we deduced that there are three ideal times to exercise on Diet Day:

1. *First thing in the morning*, eating your 100-calorie snack straight afterward;
2. *immediately before lunch*; or
3. *immediately before dinner*, if you choose dinner as your Diet Day meal.

**Exercise boosts willpower and decreases binge-ing and emotional eating.** We also found that people who dieted *and* exercised were better able to say no to extra food on Diet Day, had less tendency to overeat in response to negative emotions and binged less.

**Bottom line:** my studies show that the way to lose the *most* weight, retain the *most* calorie-burning muscle, trim the *most* tummy fat, lower LDL *and* boost HDL cholesterol levels for an optimally healthy heart and minimise self-destructive eating behaviours is by going on the Every-Other-Day Diet *and* getting regular exercise.

I want to repeat this fact – drive it home, really – because it's so important to your health and well-being: if you go on the EOD Diet *and* exercise, you will get the most benefits.

That's why I'm devoting the rest of this chapter to helping you exercise regularly.

## Are You a 'Regular' Exerciser?

What *is* 'regular exercise', exactly?

There are a lot of definitions out there and recommended levels depend on age, but guidance from the UK Chief Medical Officer for physical activity for adults is very practical and clear. Adults aged 19–64 years old should aim to be active daily, completing a minimum of 150 minutes of moderate-intensity activity (such as cycling and fast walking) or 75 minutes of vigorous-intensity activity (such as running or tennis) every week. The easiest way to approach this is to do 30 minutes of exercise at least five days a week. In addition to this activity, adults should also undertake physical activity to improve muscle strength on at least two days a week.

For more information including recommendations for other age groups see: http//www.nhs.uk/Livewell/fitness/Pages/physical-activity-guidelines-for-adults.aspx

Unfortunately, very few of us follow these guidelines. UK health surveys show only 39 per cent of men and 29 per cent of women currently meet the Chief Medical Officer's minimum recommendations for physical activity. So the obvious question is: if you're among the 60–80 per cent of under-exercisers out there – or if you're sedentary now, and need to form the exercise habit – what is the exercise you're most likely to *do*, regularly, week after week? Fortunately, there's a scientifically-proven, low-tech, easy-does-it answer to that question: walking.

A database in the USA (The National Weight Control Registry) holds lifestyle information about thousands of people who have lost at least 2 stone 2lb (13.6kg) and kept it off for at least one year. On average, those in the Registry have lost 4 stone 10lb (29.9kg) and have kept it off for 5.5 years. Among the many strategies used to lose weight and keep it off, 94 per cent of people in the Registry increased their level of physical activity, and most of them did so by *walking*. My co-author, Bill, was told this by James Hill, PhD, one of the founders of the Registry, a professor at the University of Colorado Health Sciences Center and director of the Center of Human Nutrition at the National Institutes of Health.

Walking is, of course, made up of *steps*. And many studies show the more steps you take, the less you weigh. The America On the Move study showed the average American takes only 5117 steps per day – and the fewer steps a person takes, the higher is his or her body mass index (BMI), a standard measurement of body fat.[2] A BMI of 25 to 29.9 is categorised as overweight; 30 and above is called obese. (Details of how to calculate BMI are given in chapter 1.) In the study, people who were obese walked an average of 1500 fewer steps than people who were overweight or normal weight.

In another study, from the Center for Physical Activity and Health at the University of Tennessee, people who walked an average of 10,023 steps a day had an average BMI of 24.1 – normal weight – while people who took fewer than 10,000 steps were either overweight or obese.[3]

And in a study from the Prevention Research Center at the University of South Carolina, people with an average of 9000 or more steps per day were more likely to be normal weight, while people who took fewer than 5000 steps were more likely to be obese.[4]

If you don't exercise regularly now, walking is a great way to start – and in this chapter you'll find a pedometer-based walking programme that we feel is the ideal way to start and maintain an exercise routine, particularly for people who need to lose weight. But if walking isn't for you, don't worry. The key to regular exercise, say experts, is to find a physical activity that you *enjoy* – because that's the activity you'll do regularly. Maybe it's gardening, dancing or swimming; or maybe it's a combination of different activities, which helps keep you from becoming bored.

If you're already exercising regularly, we have tips for you, too, from a leading researcher in exercise psychology who has established why people typically stop exercising (lack of willpower) and exactly what to do about it. Let's take a look at that researcher's ideas.

## FIVE SECRETS OF REGULAR EXERCISE

Is your garage or loft the Museum of Good Intentions, with dusty displays of exercise equipment and machines you ordered with enthusiasm, but used only for a few weeks or months? If so, you're far from alone. A lot of resolutions fail because of a lack of resolve or willpower, and exercising regularly is certainly one of them. Half of all people who start an exercise routine stop within six months.

But there are several strategies to make sure you *always* have enough willpower to exercise, no matter what type of exercise you choose, says Kathleen Martin Ginis, PhD, a professor of health and exercise psychology in the Department of Kinesi-ology at McMaster University in Canada.

The surprising fact is that willpower is *not* an unlimited resource, and that you have to manage and conserve it, so there's always enough when you need it.

'Willpower can weaken and then fatigue completely – just like a muscle you're using to lift weights,' Dr Martin Ginis explained. 'This "limited-strength model of willpower" – first described by Roy Baumeister, PhD, at Florida State – says that willpower is a *finite, renewable* resource that is drained when you try to control your behaviours, thoughts or emotions.' At that point, you have to *wait* for willpower to 'recover' before you can use it again, she said. And knowing how to keep the 'power' in 'willpower' can make all the difference in whether or not you exercise regularly.

Below are Dr Martin Ginis's suggestions for always having plenty of willpower to get out and exercise.

### 1. Make a plan

'This is particularly important for people starting an exercise programme,' she said. 'You have to think through where you're going to exercise, what exercise you'll do when you get there, how you'll fit the exercise into your day and what you'll do if and when the exercise starts to feel uncomfortable.'

'Because there's so much thinking and planning around exercise – all of which demand willpower – the best strategy is to plan your exercise in advance.'

'For example, at the beginning of the month, or the begin-ning of the week, take out your diary and figure out the days you'll be exercising, and the time of day you'll do it.'

'This type of advance planning removes the need for a lot of daily self-control. When the planned time for exercise rolls around, you don't have to use your limited willpower making a decision whether or not to exercise – the decision is already made. Just get up out of your chair and go.

'Planning is an astoundingly effective strategy for not draining willpower – and for maintaining regular exercise,' she said.

### 2. Exercise in the morning

This is an effective strategy for those who are morning people. 'You exercise before other activities drain willpower,' Dr Martin Ginis said.

### 3. Take a break and then exercise

'Rest is always the best way to replenish willpower,' she said. 'Take 10 to 15 minutes, close your eyes and meditate or catnap. Then go out and exercise.'

### 4. Boost your mood

'A good mood helps you muster up willpower,' she said. 'Listen to music you like. Read a joke book.'

### 5. Strengthen your willpower by using it

'If you consistently use your willpower – resisting a second piece of chocolate cake, stopping yourself from checking your email every 15 minutes, resisting the urge to hit the snooze button when your alarm goes off in the morning – you'll gradually increase the strength of your willpower, so that it more readily responds when you need it for any activity,' she said.

'Willpower is like a muscle,' she emphasised. 'Using it is temporarily draining, but builds greater strength for the next time you want to "exercise" self-control.'

Behavioural scientists say there are three more essential strategies to making a positive change in your life, such as forming and maintaining an exercise habit:

1. Set a goal.
2. Monitor yourself.
3. Relish the satisfaction of success once you reach your goal.

There's a simple device you can buy very cheaply that allows you to do those three very things: a pedometer.

## YOUR PEDOMETER-BASED WALKING PROGRAMME

A *pedometer* is a small device you clip to your belt or waistband or carry in your pocket, where it counts and displays the number of steps you take each day. Using a pedometer is like having access to a trainer who is *always* helping you maintain or increase your level of physical activity. When researchers from Stanford analysed 26 studies on pedometers and walking, involving nearly 3000 people, they found that those using a pedometer increased their daily activity by an average of nearly 2500 steps per day – a little more than 1 mile (1.6km).[5] If you're not already a regular exerciser, a pedometer-based walking programme is a great way to get started. Here's how to choose a pedometer and get going.

## THE PRIMO PEDOMETER

Ready to put on a pedometer and see where it takes you? Well, you'll quickly discover there are *hundreds* of pedometers on the market. How do you choose? Do what we did: ask a world-class pedometer expert . . .

'I recommend the Omron HJ-112, which is *very* reliable,' Dr Richardson said. 'It's accurate, durable, easy to use and cheap.' (You can find one on Amazon for £27.99.)

You can put this pedometer in your pocket or your handbag or clip it to your belt or waistband – it's accurate in *any* position. That's not the case with many other pedometers, which have to be vertical to register a step. And accuracy is crucial: you don't want a pedometer that undercounts (so you never reach your goal) or overcounts (so you think you've reached it, but you haven't).

A slightly more expensive Omron pedometer – the HJ720-ITC – has a USB port, so you can upload your steps into the accompanying software that helps you track (and reach) your goals; this is the pedometer Dr Richardson uses in all her studies on pedometers and health.

Some pedometers – like the wireless Fitbit – automatically upload your step info to a computer program or smartphone application that tracks steps. And Fitbit (and several other wireless pedometers) are compatible with the smartphone programs from www.myfitnesspal.com, that are used by hundreds of thousands of people to keep track of daily calories.

Although the Omron models are her favourites, there are many other good devices available, Dr Richardson said.

*(continued)*

'There are hundreds of new pedometers every year, with prices dropping and the quality increasing - everybody can find a pedometer that works for them.'

## Figure Out Your Daily Step Count

You've bought your pedometer and are ready to increase your steps. Don't do it – at least not for the first week. 'Wear a pedometer for seven days to determine your baseline,' said Dr Caroline Richardson, one of the world's leading experts in using pedometers for weight control and wellness, an associate professor in the Department of Family Medicine at the University of Michigan, and a researcher at the Ann Arbor Veterans Administration Center for Clinical Management Research. Here's her step-by-step method for determining your daily average of steps, or baseline:

1. Each night at bedtime, write down your steps for that day.
2. After seven days, add up the week's total of steps. (Some pedometers, like the Omron HJ-112, keep a record of the previous seven days of steps.)
3. Divide the number by 7 to get your daily average.

That figure is your baseline – and now you're ready to increase it! Add 1200 steps per day for the first week: if your baseline was 5000, your goal is to walk 6200 steps per day. 'That's enough steps to be a bit challenging, but not so many that it's impossible,' Dr Richardson said.

Then add an additional 1200 the second week (so you are at 7400 steps per day); and 1200 more the third week (so you're at 8600 per day); and so on, until you've reached 10,000 steps per day. However, Dr Richardson also advised *individualising* those increases, depending on your situation. For example, if you're obese or have a chronic disease, consider increasing your baseline by only 600 to 800 steps per day for the first week. If your baseline was 5000, your goal is to walk 5600 steps per day the first week; 6200 steps per day the second week; and so on.

'With my patients, I constantly adjust the 1200-per-day [step] number and overall number, depending on what the person can do,' she said. 'If he's not making his goal, or only half his goal, I don't add 1200 steps per week.'

How do you increase your steps week by week? The obvious way is to go for a daily walk of 30 minutes or more. Walking briskly, you can log 3000 steps in about 30 minutes. Several shorter walks – of 5, 10, or 15 minutes – are also a good strategy.

What's important is that you actually *take* those steps. When researchers in the Department of Sports Medicine at the University of Southern Maine studied 34 people involved in an eight-week 'pedometer-based lifestyle intervention', they found the walkers typically chose one or more of ten basic strategies to increase their daily steps.[6]

They walked:

- before work
- to a meeting or on a work-related errand
- using the stairs, rather than the elevator

- at lunch
- after work
- to a destination like work or the shops
- after parking farther away from a destination than usual
- with the dog
- on the weekend
- while travelling

My preference is walking to work. I take the train to and from work every day. Going to work, I get off at a station two miles away from the University of Illinois and walk the rest of the way. Coming home, I walk two miles to that same station. That's 8000 steps' worth of walking, so I know I'm meeting the 10,000-step goal every day.

Bill wears a pedometer from when he gets up in the morning to when he goes to bed at night. On at least four days a week, he logs 4–6000 steps per day by going on a walk of 45 to 60 minutes.

## STEP UP TO FITNESS – MORE IDEAS FOR GETTING EXTRA STEPS

James Hill, PhD, a professor at the University of Colorado Health Sciences Center, has plenty of ideas for how to build more steps into your day:

### At work

- Take two ten-minute walks during the day.
- Walk to the cloakroom, water dispenser, or photocopier on a different floor.

- Walk a few laps around your floor during breaks.
- Take five-minute walking breaks from your computer.
- Get off the bus earlier before work and walk the extra distance to work.
- Walk around while using a speakerphone, cordless phone or mobile phone.
- Find a lunch spot that is at least a ten-minute walk each way to/from your office.

### Out and about

- Return your shopping trolley to the designated area.
- Walk around the airport while waiting for your plane.
- Make several trips to unload your shopping from your car.
- Avoid the drive-thru – get out of your car and walk inside.
- Walk around the local shopping centre.
- Walk to your nearest postbox to post a letter, instead of dropping it off by car.
- Walk around the playing fields at your children's games.
- Pick up litter in your neighbourhood or park.

### At home with family and friends

- Walk around the living room during TV adverts. There's scientific proof to back up this idea. In a recent study conducted by researchers at the National Cancer Institute, sedentary, overweight people did 'TV Commercial Stepping' during 90 minutes of daily TV watching.[7] After six months, their average daily step

*(continued)*

count had increased from 4611 to 7605. A similar group assigned to daily walking with a pedometer increased their steps from 4909 to 7865. In other words, *both* strategies worked to increase steps.

- Go up and down the stairs with washing or other household items separately, instead of combining trips.
- Empty waste-paper baskets every day.
- Walk to a neighbour's or friend's house instead of phoning them.

## Make the Small Changes That Drive Success

If you've never exercised before, it's unrealistic to think that you're going to instantly be a marathon runner. The trick is to set realistic, achievable goals and to increase your activity in small amounts.

'Small changes drive success,' Dr Hill said. He didn't always think that way. But now he knows better.

'I spent most of my career trying to get people to make *big* lifestyle changes,' he said. 'They made them – but they didn't stick with them. I've done a total about-face in my approach to lifestyle change because now I understand that *small changes* are what work.'

How does a pedometer fit into that philosophy?

'Let me give you an example,' Dr Hill said. 'A patient of mine decides to follow the physical activity recommendations to get anywhere from 30 to 90 minutes of moderate to intense physical activity on most days of the week. Well, if he's like many of the overweight people I work with, he probably hasn't been off the couch in six months. Even 30 minutes of physical activity isn't going to be easy for him. But he's determined to give it a try. He joins a gym, works out a couple of days a week for two to three weeks – and then stops. *Why* did he stop? Because the change was too big to sustain.

'But with a pedometer, he doesn't have to achieve a big goal right away, like exercising for 30 minutes most days of the week. Instead, he determines how many steps he takes each day, and then he increases the number by a *little bit*. He moves *toward* his goal, little by little.'

Small changes allow you to get motivated and stay motivated 'until you've made a big, extraordinary change', Dr Hill said. And when you've achieved a big change, through a series of small changes, it's much more likely you'll *stay* changed.

It's also important to set a goal for yourself – for example, getting to 10,000 steps in a pedometer programme. Whatever your pace in reaching the 10,000-steps-per-day level, Dr Richardson thinks that number of daily steps is a good goal for most people – *because* it's not too easy to achieve. 'It's a challenge to reach 10,000 steps,' she said. 'You have to take a 60-minute walk per day, or a lot of little walks throughout the day. And a challenge is *good.*'

'Thousands of studies on goal-setting show that *high, hard goals* are what maximise success – and it doesn't matter how high and hard they are, as long as the person thinks there is a reasonable chance of achieving the goal. People *like* high, hard goals – they're motivating and fun.'

### Believe in Yourself

Another important part of increasing your level of physical activity is what behavioural scientists call *self-efficacy*, says Dr Richardson. You have to *believe* you can reach the goal. With a pedometer, that's easy. She gives an example:

'I tell one of my patients to increase her steps by 1000 a day. She walks down the hall and back and sees that she's just put 100 steps on her pedometer. She says to herself, "Wow, I just got 100 steps – I'm going to walk down that hall again."'

That feel-good experience is quite different from what typically happens when a well-meaning doctor tells you to 'get more exercise'.

'When you're sedentary and a doctor tells you to exercise more, you really don't know where to start,' Dr Richardson said. You might work out too hard and feel lousy afterward. And you might still feel like a failure, because you really don't know if you exercised enough. But with a pedometer, you have a concrete goal. You know exactly what you need to do and whether you've done it or not. And when you do it, you feel good about yourself.

So whether you decide to walk using a pedometer, or jog a couple of days a week, or ride an exercise bike, or you choose another type of physical activity, try to find a way to go on the Every-Other-Day Diet *and* exercise regularly. You'll lose more weight, trim more tummy fat and your heart will be that much healthier. Your body was built to move. If you're not exercising regularly now, it might be a bit hard to get moving at first. But once you do, you'll be glad you did!

## EOD – Easy as 1-2-3

1. Appreciate the unique pound-shedding power of combining the EOD Diet with regular exercise.
2. Use the Five Secrets of Regular Exercise (see p. 147) to start an exercise programme and stay on track.
3. Walk. It's the most popular form of exercise among people who successfully lose weight. Use a pedometer to help you walk regularly.

## CHAPTER 6

# The Every-Other-Day Success Programme: The Scientifically-Proven Way to Keep the Weight Off

*Five out of six dieters regain their weight; you won't be one of them*

You've probably heard the famous Mark Twain quote about quitting smoking. 'It's easy,' he said. 'I've done it hundreds of times.' Many of us could say something very similar about losing weight, and that probably includes you. If you're reading this book, it's likely you've read other diet books, tried their diets, lost weight and then gained the weight back – every single pound, every single time. Welcome to the club, which has about 100 million members.

A recent survey in the USA found that 55 per cent of American adults are currently on a weight-loss diet. But research also shows that five out of six people who diet and lose weight subsequently *regain* their weight – *all* of it, after just one year. That's right: for every six people who go on a diet and lose weight, only one is trimmer a year later. And scientists now understand why.

## THE REASONS YOU REGAIN THE WEIGHT

When you lose a lot of weight, your body's metabolism – the pace at which it burns calories – resets itself. Moment by moment, day by day, *you burn fewer calories than you did before you lost weight.*

Scientists call this phenomenon *adaptive thermogenesis.* They don't know exactly why it happens. But they do have an evolutionary theory, which could be called the Survival of the Fattest. It posits that the body has a mind of its own; when you dieted, it thought its food supply was threatened. Now it thinks it has to preserve fat for you to stay alive. So your body has decided to burn fewer calories – for the rest of your life, which it hopes is as long as possible.

Say, for example, that you weighed 17 stone 2lb (113.4kg) and lost 3 stone 8lb (22.7kg). If you compare your daily caloric needs to those of an adult who has *always* weighed 14 stone 4lb (90.7kg) – an adult who has never dieted – you, the ex-dieter, need to eat 15–25 per cent *fewer* calories to maintain the same weight. That's because the calories the ex-dieter takes in are burned much more slowly.

A moderately active man who has slimmed down to

14 stone 4lb (90.7kg) has a daily maintenance level of about 3250 calories. But post-diet, he needs to eat only about 2500 calories to maintain his weight, or *750 fewer calories per day* than a similarly active man who has always been that weight. That's nearly an entire meal less, every day!

Forgoing an entire meal every day is no picnic – literally! Five out of six of us can't do it. And five out of six of us regain the weight.

There's a second reason why weight regain is so common. During traditional dieting, you shed metabolically active, calorie-burning *muscle* along with fat, which further interferes with your ability to burn up rather than store post-diet calories. And if you regain weight, you're likely to regain most of it as *fat*, which is why many dieters don't just return to their old weight; with less muscle to burn calories, they end up heavier than ever.

Another reason you regain weight: your body doesn't only reset its metabolism after a significant weight loss to protect you from starvation. It's a lot smarter than that. It also starts to pump out a different ratio of the hormones that control your appetite. You manufacture more *ghrelin*, the hormone that *increases* hunger. You manufacture less *leptin*, the hormone that *decreases* hunger. In short, you're hungrier. And so you eat more.

## THE EVERY-OTHER-DAY SUCCESS PROGRAMME: REVERSING THE REASONS FOR REGAIN

So your metabolism has slowed to a crawl, forcing you to eat about one-third less than a non-dieter to maintain the same weight. There's a hunger hormone sitting on your shoulder like a devil, whispering, *Eat, eat, eat.* And to make matters worse, a bunch of your muscle has abandoned ship. What's a dieter to do?

Well, other diet books either ignore this rebound effect or mislead the reader about it, assuring dieters they won't regain their weight – with no scientific evidence to support their claim.

The Every-Other-Day Diet is different. I don't avoid or whitewash this issue. Instead, I offer the Every-Other-Day Success Programme – a new, every-other-day pattern of eating, similar to the diet itself, but not as low in calories. Once you reach your goal weight, you start the EOD Success Programme. And like the Every-Other-Day Diet, the Success Programme is supported by scientific research – my *newest* research, which shows that people who lose weight on the EOD Diet and then go on the Success Programme *don't* regain that weight. Before we get to those spectacular results, I'm sure you're wondering just how the Success Programme works.

## WHAT IS THE EVERY-OTHER-DAY SUCCESS PROGRAMME?

You transition to the EOD Success Programme as soon as you reach your goal weight. And the essence of the programme couldn't be simpler:

*Eat 1000 calories on Monday, Wednesday and Friday (Success Days), and eat as much as you want*

***and whatever you want on the other days of the week (Feast Days).***

My study participants were asked to limit their calories every other day, and they did – but only during the week! Most of them decided to take the weekend off. And that turned out just fine. They still maintained their weight loss and all the other healthy changes they had achieved while on the EOD Diet. (And that was OK with me. As a scientist, I'm most interested in what *really* works, not an approach I think *might* work.)

During the EOD Diet, Diet Day typically consisted of one 400-calorie meal and one 100-calorie snack. During the EOD Success Programme, Success Day consists of two 400-calorie meals and two 100-calorie snacks. You can consume those meals and snacks in any pattern of daily eating that you prefer – one large meal, three smaller meals – as long as you don't exceed 1000 calories.

Feast Days are the same as they were on the EOD Diet: eat all the food you want, and eat any food you want. However, because this is a lifelong programme, my study participants were counselled about healthy food choices and lifestyle habits to support a lifetime of weight maintenance and good health. You'll find similar information later in this chapter. But before getting to that practical info, let's take a closer look at the results of my study on the Success Programme – results that will give you the confidence you need to embark on this lifelong journey of weight maintenance.

## SPECTACULAR RESULTS IN WEIGHT LOSS *AND* IN WEIGHT MAINTENANCE

In chapter 1, I describe the results of many of the studies I've conducted on the Every-Other-Day Diet, including the results from the first year of an ongoing three-year study sponsored by the National Institutes of Health (NIH). But the NIH study is unique. It doesn't just look at the Every-Other-Day Diet. It also looks at the Every-Other-Day Success Programme.

This three-year study consists of three one-year experiments. For the first six months of the year, the participants are on the EOD Diet, *losing* weight. For the next six months they are on the Every-Other-Day Success Programme, *maintaining* weight.

I'm delighted to report (as I did in November 2013, at the annual 'ObesityWeek' conference, the world's most prestigious conference on obesity and weight loss[1]) that *both* every-other-day programmes work: on the Every-Other-Day Diet people shed pounds; and on the Every-Other-Day Success Programme people maintain that weight loss. Let's take a closer look at those results – and what they mean for *you*.

**You'll eat fewer calories automatically.** The Every-Other-Day Success Programme was originally designed to provide 50 per cent of normal calories on one day (Success Day) and 150 per cent of normal calories on the next (Feast Day). My first surprise: hardly anybody could eat 150 per cent of their Feast Day calories in a single day! The study participants topped out at an average of 125 per cent.

In other words, whatever metabolic and hormonal forces were in play, the unique effect of EOD eating stopped those former dieters from overeating. They *automatically* ate the more limited amount of calories necessary for weight maintenance!

**You'll keep losing weight – and keep it off.** If you're sitting down, stand up and cheer! Because the study results are worth celebrating.

While on the EOD Diet, the participants in the study lost from 1 stone 1lb – 3 stone 8lb (6.8–22.7kg), with an average loss of 1 stone 11lb (11.3kg). While on the EOD Success Programme, those same dieters gained back an average of 1lb. (That's right – *1lb.*)

***Bottom line:*** participants hardly regained any weight. They maintained their weight loss. Where five out of six people on other diets failed, EOD dieters succeeded. And they did that by continuing the EOD pattern: eating 1000 calories one day and all they wanted the next.

**You'll lose fat, not muscle.** As I pointed out previously, people lose 75 per cent fat and 25 per cent muscle on a typical diet, and shedding all that muscle sabotages the ability to maintain weight loss. In this study, as in all of my previous studies on the Every-Other-Day Diet, the participants shed most of their weight as fat, and very little as muscle.

Taking the average weight loss of 1 stone 11lb (11.3kg):

- 1 stone 9lb (10.4kg) of that was fat;
- 2lb (0.9kg) was muscle

That's a big reason why the Every-Other-Day Success Programme *is* a success.

**You'll bust tummy fat, big-time.** The EOD Diet whittled

away the waistlines of the study participants, with an average decrease of more than 5" (12.7cm). (The men lost more abdominal fat than the women, because they had more to begin with.) And that extra fat wasn't regained on the Success Programme:

- Abdominal fat lost on the EOD Diet: 2–6lb (0.9–2.7kg)
- Abdominal fat regained on the EOD Success Programme: none
- Average waistline reduced on the EOD Diet: 5½" (14cm)
- Average waistline regained on the EOD Success Programme: nothing

Trimming tummy fat does more than boost your self-esteem and help you get back into your skinny jeans. A bulging abdomen is the outward sign of excess *visceral* fat, the 'deep' fat that wraps around your inner organs and ruins your health. Every extra pound of visceral fat translates into higher risk for heart disease, stroke and type-2 diabetes. Likewise, every pound you lose lowers your risk.

**You'll continue to protect your heart.** In my NIH study, participants lowered their LDL cholesterol by an average of 11 per cent during the diet, and that decrease continued during the Success Programme. They lowered their blood pressure by an average of 9 points, and that drop continued during the Success Programme. They decreased their fasting glucose by 8 per cent (high glucose is a risk factor for both heart disease and type-2 diabetes), and that decrease continued during the Success Programme.

As you can see, both the Every-Other-Day Diet and the Every-Other-Day Success Programme *work*.

- You lose weight and don't regain it.
- You lose fat (but not muscle), and the fat stays away.
- You trim inches off your waistline, and they don't inch back.
- LDL cholesterol drops and stays down.
- Blood pressure lowers and stays lower.
- Glucose levels fall and don't go back up.

---

### VICTORIA'S STORY: 'IT WILL BE EASY TO CONTROL MY WEIGHT FOR THE REST OF MY LIFE'

*Weight loss: 1 stone 13lb (12.2kg)*

A medical technician and Chicago resident, 33-year-old, 5'5" (1.7m) Victoria weighed 17 stone 7lb (111.1kg), until she went on the Every-Other-Day Diet.

'I have two school-age children and a full-time job, and I'm very busy, without much time to cook,' she said. 'Before going on the diet, I ate whatever I wanted to – fast foods, fried foods, just grabbing something on the go.'

The Every-Other-Day Diet helped her slow down a bit and plan a lot of meals for both herself and her kids, both on Diet Day and on Feast Day, and she slowly but surely began to shed pounds, hitting 15 stone 8lb (98.9kg).

When we talked to her, she had been on the Every-Other-Day Success Programme for a few months and had lost 1 stone 13lb (12.2kg). 'I'm *still* losing 1–2lb (0.5–0.9kg) per week, compared to the 2–3lb (0.9–1.4kg) per week while I was on the diet,' she said. 'I just mimic what I did on the diet.'

*(continued)*

On Success Day, she controls her hunger by drinking tea and chewing gum. She also enjoys eating the same ready meals she ate on Diet Day because they taste good and are convenient, but now she can have two main meals instead of one.

On Feast Day, Victoria has started to eat more fresh food, such as salads, steamed vegetables and fruit. And she's exercising regularly, working out two or three times a week.

Victoria is very intent on success because she's dieted before, lost the weight and has *always* regained it.

'Success Day is very important to me because I want to keep the weight off,' she said. 'With other diets, they lasted a few months, and that's it. With the Every-Other-Day Success Programme, it will be easy to control my weight for the rest of my life – and that's what I'm going to do!'

## Keep Up the Good Work!

There are a lot of habits I recommended that you start while on the EOD Diet, to help you maximise weight loss and good health, and I hope you keep on doing them! We'll review them below.

*Get regular exercise.* In chapter 5, I discussed the power of combining the Every-Other-Day Diet with regular exercise and introduced you to a pedometer-based walking programme. If you started walking (or doing any other type of regular exercise) while on the EOD Diet, congratulations – don't stop now! Here's why. A register in the USA of thousands of people who have lost weight and kept it off for at least one year shows that 94 per cent of them increased their physical activity level. Most of them did so by walking.

And when researchers at Harvard Medical School studied more than 4500 women aged 26 to 45 who had lost weight, they found that those who added just 30 minutes of physical activity to their daily routine (brisk walking was a favourite) were 52 per cent less likely to regain a lot of weight in the two years after they shed the pounds.[2]

If you haven't read chapter 5 – 'Every-Other-Day Dieting and Exercise' – I strongly encourage you to do so. And I also strongly encourage you to do what that chapter says to do: exercise regularly, using either the pedometer-based walking programme described in the chapter or some other form of exercise.

***Weigh yourself every day.*** Studies show this habit not only helps with weight loss, but also with weight mainte-nance, as we discussed earlier (see p. 44). If, for whatever reason, you see the pounds creeping back on, go back on the EOD Diet until you've returned to your goal weight – and then restart the Success Programme.

***Drink plenty of water.*** Drinking an 8-ounce (227ml) glass of water 15 or 30 minutes before each meal is a great way to control hunger and calorie intake on Success Day, as we discussed earlier (see p. 64). Drinking water throughout the day also helps.

***Chew gum.*** This is another simple habit that can improve your chances of long-term weight maintenance. It cuts hun-ger and appetite and increases alertness. It even burns a few extra calories.

## CALORIE COUNTING MADE EASY

There are a lot of different ways to take in the 1000 calories of Success Day – one, two or three meals, and one or two snacks. Any combination works, as long as you don't exceed the calorie limit. What's the best way to keep track of those calories? Let me count the ways you can count the calories.

*Use chapter 4.* You can prepare the calorie-controlled recipes and snacks from chapter 4: one 400-calorie lunch, one 400-calorie dinner, and two 100-calorie snacks to total 1000 calories. Or choose ready meals that add up to 1000 calories.

*Buy cookbooks featuring meals of 400 or fewer calories.* For more recipes, you can also buy and use one or more of the many cookbooks that offer 400- and 500-calorie meals and 100-calorie snacks. Some of our favourites: *400 Calorie Fix Cookbook*; *EatingWell 500-Calorie Dinners*; *Mix & Match Low-Calorie Cookbook* from CookingLight (the breakfast and lunch recipes are under 400 calories, and the dinner recipes are under 500); *500 400-Calorie Recipes*; the *400 Calorie* series from Good Housekeeping (which includes a general cookbook and cookbooks featuring chicken, Italian, vegetarian, and comfort foods); *The Complete Idiot's Guide to 200-300-400 Calorie Meals*; and *The 100-Calorie Snack Cookbook*.

*Google '400-calorie recipes'.* You'll get more than 8 million results!

*Download a calorie-counting app or buy a calorie coun-ter.* Use a smartphone app for calorie-counting, like Calorie Counter by Fat Secret, My Meal Mate or MyFitnessPal. Apps are particularly efficient for calorie counting: they're always with you and they're easy to use. You can also go the old-fashioned route and buy a book to help you with calorie-counting. One of the most popular is *The Calorie, Carb & Fat Bible 2013: The UK's Most Comprehensive Calorie Counter* by Costain, Kellow and Beeken.

*Use the calorie cheat sheet (below) of food categories as a guide.* An interesting and helpful way to think about calories is to think of foods in terms of *calories per pound*, advises Jeffrey Novick, MS, RD, a dietitian and nutritionist in California who has worked with Whole Foods in developing their Wellness Club. Of course, you wouldn't eat a pound of broccoli or a pound of butter. But a pound-for-pound comparison between the two foods shows just how many calories each packs and the differences between them – and why emphasising vegetables, fresh fruits, whole grains, legumes and lean proteins can help you stay within the 1000-calorie limit of Success Day. Here is a list of some food categories and their calories per pound (0.5kg), in general:

- *Vegetables:* 100 to 200 calories per pound of food
- *Fresh fruits:* 200 to 300 calories per pound of food
- *Whole grains and legumes:* 500 calories per pound of food

*(continued)*

- *Lean proteins, like seafood and the white meat of chicken:* 600 to 650 calories per pound of food
- *Fattier proteins, like a steak served at a restaurant specialising in 'premium' steaks:* 1000 calories per pound of food
- *Refined, processed carbohydrates, such as breads, bagels and crackers:* 1200 to 1500 calories per pound of food
- *Junk food, such as sugary biscuits made with white flour:* 2000 calories per pound of food
- *Nuts and seeds:* 2800 calories per pound of food
- *Oils and fats:* 4000 calories per pound of food

Not to worry: calorie counting isn't for ever. If you're like most people, you tend to eat the same one or two dozen foods over and over. After two to three months, you won't need any assistance in knowing how many calories you're taking in; it will be obvious to you.

## MINDFUL EATING AND PORTION CONTROL: TWO OTHER KEYS TO WEIGHT MAINTENANCE

In addition to the tips we've already given you in this book, I want to discuss two others that will go a long way toward helping you maintain your weight loss.

Maintaining your weight loss isn't just about *what* you eat. It's also about *why* you eat. And what you do *when* you eat. Maybe there are times when you eat not because you feel *hungry*, but because you feel *lousy*. You use food to tranquillise negative emotions, ease stress or relieve boredom. Maybe there are food 'cues' that you always respond to – see a biscuit, eat it – whether you're hungry or not.

And maybe there are times (maybe even most of the time) when you don't pay attention to the smell and taste and sensual enjoyment of eating. Instead, you eat in a rush – in the car or in front of the TV – barely noticing the food.

Research links these three habits – what scientists call *emotional eating, external eating* and *distracted eating* – to overweight and obesity. But there's a habit that's pretty much the exact *opposite* of emotional, distracted and external eating. And many studies, as I'll describe in a moment, link this habit to successful weight maintenance. It's called *mindful eating.*

Mindful eating is being aware of your emotions and moods in the moment – not judging them, not trying to get rid of them, just *observing* and *accepting* them – and therefore not letting anxiety, depression, boredom or stress compel you to eat when you're not hungry.

Mindful eating is not letting old habits rule your life, but instead taking a step back – paying attention to your hunger and desires in the present moment – and deciding whether or not you *really* want those biscuits. And even if you do decide to eat them, maybe you decide to eat just one or two, and not the whole packet.

Mindful eating is paying attention to eating when you're eating. You notice the smell, taste and texture of the food, and you eat slowly enough to *enjoy* it. You don't do anything else while you eat. Mindful eating is having an *intention* – maintaining your weight loss – and then having the *attention* to accomplish it.

I think mindful eating is one of the most powerful and important aids to success on the Every-Other-Day Success Programme. The participants in my NIH-sponsored study were taught the skill. Plus, there's a lot of scientific research supporting the role of mindful eating in controlling weight. Some recent studies found the following:

***If you're distracted, you eat more – a lot more.*** When a team of UK researchers analysed studies on 'eating attentively', they found that people who were distracted during eating ate a lot more food – up to 76 per cent more than people who were attentive while eating. 'Attentive eating is likely to influence food intake,' wrote the researchers in the *American Journal of Clinical Nutrition.*[3]

***If you eat mindfully, you eat smaller portions of high-calorie foods.*** In a study of 171 people published in the scientific journal *Appetite*, those who were more 'mindful eaters' ate smaller portions of high-calorie foods.[4]

***If you're mindful, you have fewer cravings and do less emotional eating.*** In a study by Dutch researchers, 26 women took a training course in mindful eating and as a result had fewer food cravings, and did less emotional and external eating. 'Mindfulness practice can be an effective way to reduce . . . problematic eating behavior,' wrote the researchers in *Appetite.*[5]

***When you're mindful, your brain is less preoccupied with food!*** Researchers at Wake Forest University School of Medicine conducted brain scans (functional magnetic resonance imaging, or fMRI) on 19 obese people after they ate breakfast and weren't allowed to eat again for nearly three hours. Those with more mindfulness had 'greater . . .

efficiency' in their 'brain networks', indicating they were less preoccupied with eating again.[6]

***Mindfulness = weight maintenance.*** Researchers at the Osher Center for Integrative Medicine at the University of California, San Francisco, studied 47 overweight and obese women, dividing them into two groups. One group received mindfulness training aimed at reducing 'stress eating' and one group didn't. After four months, the mindful group was less anxious, had less external-based eating, pumped out less of the stress hormone cortisol and maintained their weight. Meanwhile, the non-mindful group gained weight.[7]

## How to be a mindful eater

One of the top experts on mindful eating is Michelle May, MD, founder and CEO of the Am I Hungry? Mindful Eating Workshops, and author of *Eat What You Love, Love What You Eat* and several other books on mindful eating. Here are some of the key principles of mindful eating that Dr May has shared with Bill. We'd like to note that Dr May does not endorse the Every-Other-Day Diet, the Every-Other-Day Success Programme, or any other weight-loss programme or diet. But because her recommendations about mindful eating are uniquely insightful and effective, we wanted to share them with you.

***Before you eat, ask yourself: 'Why am I eating?'*** 'People eat for reasons other than hunger,' Dr May said. 'Often the cues are emotional, such as loneliness, depression, anxiety, stress or boredom. These cues override our *internal* cues of hunger and fullness, and send you in the direction of comforting, convenient and calorie-dense foods. And because you're not hungry when you *start* to eat, you don't know when to stop. You eat until the food is gone.

'Instead,' she says, 'ask yourself this simple question before you eat: "Why am I eating?"'

'Put a speed bump – a pause – between wanting to eat and starting to eat. Take a moment to realise what's really going on, whether you're physically hungry or responding to an emotional cue. If you discover you're not hungry, make a choice whether to use food to deal with something that isn't a physical need for food or to redirect your attention to something else until you're actually hungry.'

***Learn to recognise the physical signs of hunger.*** How can you tell whether or not you're hungry? *Scan* your body – particularly your stomach – for physical signs, Dr May advises. 'Get quiet for a moment,' she said. 'Scan your body from head to toe. Look for clues that your desire to eat isn't hunger, such as tension in your body, or pain or worried thoughts. Also look for clues that your desire to eat *is* hunger, like a hollow or empty feeling in your stomach, or rumbling and growling. Do this scan whenever you feel like eating, and also about every three hours throughout the day, to see if you're truly hungry and need to eat.'

***Redirect your attention.*** If you're not hungry, one strategy is to distract yourself rather than eat, Dr May said. Go for a walk. Play with your dog. Take a shower. Brush your teeth. Do your nails. Or, if you've identified the underlying emotional need that you're looking for food to satisfy, meet the need instead, in a small way. 'Maybe you're overworked and stressed out and need a vacation,' Dr May said. 'Take a few minutes to surf online and look at a travel site, or visualise being on vacation and resting in a hammock, or take a few deep breaths.'

***Learn to recognise when you feel full.*** Being able to decide not to eat when you're not hungry is one feature of mindful eating. Deciding to stop eating when you're comfortably full is another.

'Mindful eating is not about *being good* but about *feeling good*,' said Dr May. 'Identify signs of fullness and stop when you feel comfortable. A smart idea for figuring out when you're full: set an intention before you eat. Ask yourself, "How do I want to feel when I'm done?" You probably want to feel good, energetic and satisfied, not bad, tired and stuffed,' Dr May said.

## PORTION SIZES: DON'T SUPERSIZE YOURSELF

There's another habit that's probably every bit as important as mindful eating: *controlling portion size*. In fact, many nutritional scientists think the trend toward ever-bigger portions – in supermarkets, restaurants, convenience stores, at home, and even in cookbooks – is *the* main reason why so many of us have become overweight or obese. There's a lot of evidence supporting that perspective. For example, researchers in the Department of Nutrition at the University of North Carolina at Chapel Hill analysed 30 years of scientific data to find out *why* Americans were eating 600 more calories per day in 2006 than they were in 1977. They discovered two main reasons: the increase in portion sizes; and the increase in the number of times per day people eat and drink.[8] During those 30 years, the average amount of food/drink consumed per 'eating occasion' increased by 2.3oz (65g) per occasion. And those extra ounces add up pounds more quickly than ever, because there was also an average of 4.9 eating occasions per day in 2006, compared to 3.8 in 1977.

A few other alarming facts, courtesy of Brian Wansink, PhD, a professor at Cornell University and author of *Mindless Eating: Why We Eat More Than We Think*:[9]

- Jumbo-sized portions in restaurants, where we now spend more and more of our food budget, are consistently 250 per cent larger than regular portions. (And most items in fast-food restaurants are 2 to 5 times larger than they were 20 years ago, says the USDA.)
- People tend to eat 30–50 per cent more from larger-sized restaurant portions, and 20–40 per cent more from larger-sized packets. And eating a big portion today doesn't mean you'll turn one down tomorrow. In one study, normal and overweight people were served 50 per cent larger portions over a period of 11 days and they overate day after day, for a grand total of 4636 extra calories.
- The sizes of the glasses and bowls in our kitchens have steadily increased, and are now 36 per cent larger than they were in 1960.

There are two main reasons why all of this supersizing causes us to overeat, according to Dr Wansink:

- Larger packets, restaurant portions and tableware have set a 'consumption norm' that says it's 'more appropriate, typical, reasonable and normal' to eat larger portions.
- Large portions confuse us about how much we've actually eaten – you can eat a lot of food before you notice the amount has decreased! In one study, people ate 73 per cent more tomato soup from bowls that were being secretly and imperceptibly refilled from underneath the table, compared to people eating from normal bowls – while estimating they ate only 5 calories more!

The Every-Other-Day Success Programme helps you control portions by alternating the 1000-calorie modified fast of Success Day with Feast Day – you don't overeat automatically. But to limit those portions can't hurt.

### Science-based tips for portion control

Bill and I reviewed the last decade of studies on portion control to find the best, scientifically-proven ways to help you manage portions on Success Day and Feast Day:

*Use your plate to control your portions.* Researchers at the Mayo Clinic studied 65 obese people, dividing them into two groups. For six months, one group used a 'portion-control plate' for their meals; they lost nearly five times more weight than those who did not use the plates.[10] In a similar six-month study, published in the *Archives of Internal Medicine*, obese people with type-2 diabetes using portion control plates lost 18 times more weight than a similar group not using the plates.[11]

In the Mayo study, the plate was clear glass with black print that divided it into three parts: one half was labelled 'vegetables'; one quarter was labelled 'fish, lean meat, chicken and nuts'; and one quarter was labelled 'potatoes, pasta, rice, beans and whole grains'. The study participants were instructed to use the plate for their main meal and encouraged to use it for every meal.

I think dividing your meals into half vegetables and fruits, a quarter protein, and a quarter starch is a great (and easy) way to control your portions. Those portion sizes also match the latest recommendations from the USDA, where 'myplate' has replaced the food pyramid as the government's main nutritional advice. (The USDA also recommends several daily servings of low-fat dairy, and I think that's also a helpful strategy for weight maintenance.)

You don't even have to *imagine* the portions: you can buy portion-control plates like the kind used in the Mayo study (visit http://www.thedietplate.com).

***Increase the portion of fruits and vegetables.*** If you want to lower your calories, increase the portion of vegetables and fruits and decrease the portions of protein and starchy carbohydrates. A study from researchers at Pennsylvania State University published in the *American Journal of Clinical Nutrition* showed that slightly increasing vegetables and slightly decreasing protein/starch decreased the overall calories of a meal by 14 per cent.[12]

***Serve food from smaller bowls.*** When people used a large bowl to serve pasta, they served 77 per cent more than when using a medium-sized bowl, reported Dutch researchers in the *Journal of Nutrition Education and Behavior.*[13]

In a similar study, people given large bowls (2.1lb/963g) and large ice-cream scoops (3oz/85g) served themselves 53 per cent more ice cream than those given medium-sized bowls (1.1lb/482g) and medium scoops (2oz/57g).

And when cinema-goers were given free medium-sized or large buckets of popcorn to eat during the movie, those with the large buckets ate 51 per cent more popcorn.

***Buy smaller packets.*** 'A shopper can buy smaller sizes, or create their own single-portion servings by subdividing the bargain-size bag into smaller ones,' writes Dr Wansink. During mealtime, keep the large packets or containers off the table and out of sight, he adds. That goes for drinks, too, of course. Research shows we get 21 per cent of our daily calories from drinks, nearly *double* the amount in 1965.

***Buy smaller snacks.*** People given 100-calorie snacks for a week ate 841 fewer calories from snacks compared to those given standard-size snacks, reported researchers from the University of Colorado.[14]

***Order less at restaurants, or take some home.*** In one study, increasing a restaurant's portion size of pasta by one-third increased calorie intake by 43 per cent, adding 172 more calories. 'These results support the suggestion that large restaurant portions may be contributing to the obesity epidemic,' wrote the researchers in *Obesity Research*.[15]

Don't count on well-meaning chefs to protect you. A study by researchers at Clemson University, published in *Obesity*, found that the majority of 300 executive chefs believed 'large portions are a problem for weight control'. Seventy-six per cent of those chefs also claimed portions in their restaurants were 'normal'. But the researchers found that the portions of steak and pasta the chefs were actually serving were two to four times larger than the healthy portion sizes recommended by the government.[16]

What to do? 'Consider splitting an entrée, or ordering an appetiser as your entrée, or having half the dinner packaged to go,' advises Dr Wansink.

***Eat bigger portions of high-volume, low-calorie foods.*** Decreasing portion size by 25 per cent led to a decreased mealtime intake of 231 calories in a meal, reported researchers from Pennsylvania State University. But so did *increasing* the portions of low-calorie, high-volume foods, like fruits, vegetables, soups and low-fat milk – all of which allow you to eat and drink big portions of food *without* getting a lot of extra calories. 'Reductions in both portion size and energy [calorie] density can help to moderate energy intake,' wrote the researchers in the *American Journal of Clinical Nutrition*.[17]

***Go to bed – you'll eat smaller portions tomorrow!*** Yes, getting enough sleep may mean eating smaller portions. In a study from Sweden, people who got less sleep chose breakfast portions that were 14 per cent larger and mid-morning snacks that were 16 per cent larger, compared to those who had a good night's sleep.[18]

These changes and the diet and lifestyle tips in this chapter are for a *lifetime* of good health. No need to rush! If you make these changes slowly, you'll make them successfully. And you'll be rewarded by the intense satisfaction of being one of the few dieters who have lost weight and kept it off!

## BARBARA'S STORY

*Weight loss: 1 stone 7lb (9.5kg)*

The campus of the University of Illinois-Chicago borders the Veterans Administration (VA) Medical Center, and a lot of VA nurses see the leaflets advertising my studies and enrol in them; this included Barbara.

'People think nurses should know *everything* about health, but that's not how it is,' she said with a smile. 'I was sick, I was taking prednisone, I had gone up three dress sizes – and I just couldn't seem to make up my mind to stay on a diet. Then I saw the leaflet for one of Dr Varady's studies on alternate-day fasting and weight loss, and I decided that was for me.'

After three months on the Every-Other-Day Diet, Barbara had lost 1 stone 7lb (9.5kg). And she's kept it off – for 12 months.

'On Feast Day, I know I can eat anything – but I emphasise fruits and vegetables,' she said. 'My family knows I love fruit, and there's more fruit in the house than we ever had – melons, grapefruit, oranges, pomegranates, you name it.'

She's also stopped eating fried foods, which she loved. 'Now we cook a lot of food on the grill, even grilling vegetables and corn,' she said.

And she started to walk. 'I wear a pedometer and always take the stairs, and my office is on the fifth floor. And because the VA Medical Center is such a large place, I often walk between buildings, so it's not hard to get thousands of steps.

*(continued)*

'I cheat sometimes on Success Day, but not often and never on two Success Days in a row,' she said. 'That's because my biggest fear is that I'll put the weight on again, so I do what I have to do to make sure that doesn't happen. I enjoy the compliments, and how good I feel and my sense of accomplishment for having lost the weight and kept it off.'

## THE KEY WORD IN THE EOD SUCCESS PROGRAMME IS *SUCCESS!*

Whether you bought this book to lose those last 5 or 10 pounds or an extra 20, 30, 40 or more; whether you've never dieted before or failed at every diet you've tried, I know you're going to find success with both the Every-Other-Day Diet and the Every-Other-Day Success Programme. And I know it the way a scientist knows: because my careful, repeated studies show that the weight-loss and the weight-maintenance programmes described in *The Every-Other-Day Diet* actually *work*.

The Every-Other-Day Diet works to help you lose weight – whatever your weight-loss goal, I know you'll reach it!

The Every-Other-Day Success Programme works to help you keep the weight off – if you follow the programme, I know you won't regain the pounds you shed.

It's been my pleasure to bring the EOD Diet and Success Programme from the pages of scientific journals to the pages of this book, and into your life. Bill and I wish you the best, for a trim and healthy life!

## EOD - Easy as 1-2-3!

1. On the EOD Success Programme, you eat 1000 calories on Monday, Wednesday and Friday, and you eat whatever you want the other days of the week.
2. Mindful eating - slowing down and paying attention to your meal, bite by bite - is a proven key to weight maintenance.
3. Portion control - at home and wherever else you eat - is one of the best ways to control calories.

# Acknowledgments

*From Dr Krista Varady:*

I would like to thank my co-author, Bill Gottlieb, literary agent, Chris Tomasino and editor, Christine Pride, for all of their hard work, support and encouragement throughout this process. I am also grateful to Peter Jones and Marc Hellerstein for their outstanding mentorship during my doctoral and post-doctoral degrees. Last, I would like to thank my doctoral students – Surabhi Bhutani, Monica Klempel, Cynthia Kroeger, John Trepanowski and Kristin Hoddy – for their diligent work in coordinating all of the human trials discussed in this book.

*From Bill Gottlieb:*

A finished book is an occasion for expressing a lot of gratitude because so many people (too many to thank here!) have contributed to its creation and completion. But special thanks must go to . . .

My co-author, Dr Krista Varady, for her groundbreaking research, lively intelligence and constant collegiality: Krista, you were the perfect collaborator! To Stephanie Karpinske, for her excellent (and fast!) work in producing the recipes for the book, and for providing an abundance of advice about frozen foods. To Christine Tomasino, my literary agent of 15 years, who has brought her creativity, energy, canny negotiating and consistent care to each of the 15 books I've written: Chris, I can't thank you enough. To our literary lawyer, Heather Florence, for all her careful, crucial, protective work on behalf of this project. To Matt Inman, our acquisition editor at Hyperion Books; and to Liz Gough, our acquisition editor at Hodder. To Christine Pride, our superb editor, who worked at super-speed, with super-skill, and improved the book immeasurably. To Gretchen Young at Hachette, for all her diligence and kindness; thank you for making sure the manuscript kept moving! And a final thank you to all the other members of the editorial team at Hachette who brought their unique skills to producing this book.

# Notes

## Chapter 1

1. Gardner, C. D. et al., 'Comparison of the Atkins, Zone, Ornish, and LEARN Diets for Change in Weight and Related Risk Factors among Overweight Premenopausal Women: The A TO Z Weight Loss Study: A Randomized Trial', *Journal of the American Medical Association* 297, no. 9 (7 March 2007): pp.969–77.
2. Heilbronn, L. K. et al., 'Alternate-Day Fasting in Nonobese Subjects: Effects on Body Weight, Body Composition, and Energy Metabolism', *American Journal of Clinical Nutrition* 81, no. 1 (January 2005): pp.69–73.
3. Varady, K. A. et al., 'Short-Term Modified Alternate-Day Fasting: A Novel Dietary Strategy for Weight Loss and Cardioprotection in Obese Adults', *American Journal of Clinical Nutrition* 90 (2009): pp.1138–43.
4. Ibid.
5. Klempel, M. C. et al., 'Dietary and Physical Activity Adaptations to Alternate Day Modified Fasting: Implications for Optimal Weight Loss', *Nutrition Journal* 9 (2010): p.35.
6. Bhutani, S. et al., 'Improvements in Coronary Heart Disease Risk Indicators by Alternate-Day Fasting Involve Adipose Tissue Modulations', *Obesity* 18, no. 11 (November 2010): pp.2152–59.
7. Klempel, M. C. et al., 'Alternate Day Fasting (ADF) with a High-Fat Diet Produces Similar Weight Loss and Cardio-Protection as

ADF with a Low-Fat Diet', *Metabolism* 62, no. 1 (January 2013): pp.137–43.

8. Bhutani, S. et al., 'Alternate Day Fasting and Endurance Exercise Combine to Reduce Body Weight and Favorably Alter Plasma Lipids on Obese Humans', *Obesity* (14 February 2013).

9. Kramer, F. M. et al., 'Long-Term Follow-Up of Behavioral Treatment for Obesity: Patterns of Weight Regain Among Men and Women', *International Journal of Obesity* 13, no. 2 (1989): pp.123–36.

## Chapter 2

1. VanWormer, J. J. et al., 'Self-Weighing Promotes Weight Loss for Obese Adults', *American Journal of Preventive Medicine* 36, no. 1 (January 2009): pp.70–73.

2. VanWormer, J. J. et al., 'Self-Weighing Frequency is Associated with Weight Gain Prevention Over 2 Years Among Working Adults', *International Journal of Behavioral Medicine* 19, no. 3 (September 2012): pp.351–58.

3. Steinberg, D. M. et al., 'The Efficacy of a Daily Self-Weighing Weight Loss Intervention Using Smart Scales and Email', *Obesity* (20 March 2013).

4. Butryn, M. L. et al., 'Consistent Self-Monitoring of Weight: A Key Component of Successful Weight Loss Maintenance', *Obesity* 15, no. 12 (December 2007): pp.3091–96.

5. Linde, J. A. et al., 'Self-Weighing in Weight Gain Prevention and Weight Loss Trials'. *Annals of Behavioral Medicine* 30, no. 3 (December 2005): pp.210–16.

6. Douglas, S. M. et al., 'Low, Moderate, or High Protein Yogurt Snacks on Appetite Control and Subsequent Eating in Healthy Women', *Appetite* 60, no. 1 (January 2013): pp.117–22.

7. Leidy, H. J. et al., 'The Influence of Higher Protein Intake and Greater Eating Frequency on Appetite Control in Overweight and Obese Men', *Obesity* 18, no. 9 (September 2010): pp.1725–32.

8. Mozaffarian, D. et al., 'Plasma Phospholipid Long-Chain ω-3 Fatty Acids and Total and Cause-Specific Mortality in Older Adults: A Cohort Study', *Annals of Internal Medicine* 158, no. 7 (April 2013): pp.515–25.

9. Estruch, R. et al., 'Primary Prevention of Cardiovascular Disease with a Mediterranean Diet', *New England Journal of Medicine* 368, no. 14 (April 2013): pp.1279–90.

10. Siri-Tarino, P. W. et al., 'Meta-Analysis of Prospective Cohort Studies Evaluating the Association of Saturated Fat with Cardiovascular Disease', *American Journal of Clinical Nutrition* 91, no. 3 (March 2010): pp.535–46.

11. Kong, A. et al., 'Associations between Snacking and Weight Loss and Nutrient Intake Among Postmenopausal Overweight to Obese Women in a Dietary Weight-Loss Intervention', *Journal of the American Dietetic Association* 111, no. 12 (December 2011): pp.1898–903.

12. Hibi, M., et al., 'Nighttime Snacking Reduces Whole Body Fat Oxidation and Increases LDL Cholesterol in Healthy Young Women', *American Journal of Physiology: Regulatory, Integrative and Comparative Physiology* 304, no. 2 (January 2013): pp.R94–R101.

13. Stroebele, N. et al., 'Do Calorie-Controlled Portion Sizes of Snacks Reduce Energy Intake?' *Appetite* 52, no. 3 (June 2009): pp.793–6.

14. Zizza, C. A. and B. Xu, 'Snacking Is Associated with Overall Diet Quality Among Adults', *Journal of the Academy of Nutrition and Dietetics* 112, no. 2 (February 2012): pp.291–6.

15. Zizza, C. A. et al., 'Contribution of Snacking to Older Adults' Vitamin, Carotenoid, and Mineral Intakes', *Journal of the American Dietetic Association* 110, no. 5 (May 2010): pp.768–72.

16. Bachman, J. L. et al., 'Eating Frequency is Higher in Weight Loss Maintainers and Normal-Weight Individuals Than in Overweight Individuals'. *Journal of the American Dietetic Association* 111, no. 11 (November 2011): pp.1730–34.

17. Van Walleghen, E. L. et al., 'Pre-Meal Water Consumption Reduces Meal Energy Intake in Older But Not Younger Subjects', *Obesity* 15, no. 1 (January 2007): pp.93–9.

18. Davy, B. M. et al., 'Water Consumption Reduces Energy Intake at a Breakfast Meal in Obese Older Adults', *Journal of the American Dietetic Association* 108, no. 7 (July 2008): pp.1236–9.

19. Boschmann, M. et al., 'Water Drinking Induces Thermogenesis through Osmosensitive Mechanisms', *Journal of Clinical Endocrinology and Metabolism* 92, no. 8 (August 2007): pp.3334–7.

20. Akers, J. D. et al., 'Daily Self-Monitoring of Body Weight, Step Count, Fruit/Vegetable Intake, and Water Consumption: A Feasible and Effective Long-Term Weight Loss Maintenance Approach', *Journal of the Academy of Nutrition and Dietetics* 112, no. 5 (May 2012): pp.685–92.

21. Rudenga, K. J. et al., 'Amygdala Response to Sucrose Consumption is Inversely Related to Artificial Sweetener Use', *Appetite* 58, no. 2 (April 2012): pp.504–7.

22. Fowler, S. P. et al., 'Fueling the Obesity Epidemic? Artificially Sweetened Beverage Use and Long-Term Weight Gain', *Obesity* 16, no. 8 (August 2008): pp.1894–900.

23. Bernstein, A. M. et al., 'Soda Consumption and the Risk of Stroke in Men and Women', *American Journal of Clinical Nutrition* 95, no. 5 (May 2012): pp.1190–99.

24. Schernhammer, E. S. et al., 'Consumption of Artificial Sweetener- and Sugar-Containing Soda and Risk of Lymphoma and Leukemia in Men and Women', *American Journal of Clinical Nutrition* 96, no. 6 (December 2012): pp.1419–28.

25. Nettleton, J. A. et al., 'Diet Soda Intake and Risk of Incident Metabolic Syndrome and Type 2 Diabetes in the Multi-Ethnic Study of Atherosclerosis (MESA)', *Diabetes Care* 32, no. 4 (April 2009): pp.688–94.

26. Karalius, V. P. et al., 'Dietary Sugar and Artificial Sweetener Intake and Chronic Kidney Disease: A Review', *Advances in Chronic Kidney Disease* 20, no. 2 (March 2013): pp.157–64.

27. Pepino, M. Y. et al., 'Sucralose Affects Glycemic and Hormonal Responses to an Oral Glucose Load', *Diabetes Care* (30 April 2013).

28. Gavrieli, A. et al., 'Effect of Different Amounts of Coffee on Dietary Intake and Appetite of Normal-Weight and Overweight/Obese Individuals', *Obesity* (29 November 2012).

29. Lopez-Garcia, E. et al., 'Changes in Caffeine Intake and Long-Term Weight Change in Men and Women', *American Journal of Clinical Nutrition* 83, no. 3 (March 2006): pp.674–80.

30. Carter, B. E. et al., 'Beverages Containing Soluble Fiber, Caffeine, and Green Tea Catechins Suppress Hunger and Lead to Less Energy Consumption at the Next Meal', *Appetite* 59, no. 3 (December 2012): pp.755–61.

31. Hursel, R. et al., 'The Effects of Green Tea on Weight Loss and Weight Maintenance: A Meta-Analysis', *International Journal of Obesity* 33, no. 9 (September 2009): pp.956–61.

32. Freedman, N. D. et al., 'Association of Coffee Drinking with Total and Cause-Specific Mortality', *New England Journal of Medicine* 366, no. 20 (May 2012): pp.1891–904.

33. Hetherington, M. M. et al., 'Effects of Chewing Gum on Short-Term Appetite Regulation in Moderately Restrained Eaters', *Appetite* 57, no. 2 (October 2011): pp.475–82.

34. Smith, A. P. et al., 'Effects of Chewing Gum on the Stress and Work of University Students', *Appetite* 58, no. 3 (June 2012): pp.1037–40.

35. Zibell, S. et al., 'Impact of Gum Chewing on Stress Levels: Online Self-Perception Research Study', *Current Medical Research and Opinion* 25, no. 6 (June 2009): pp.1491–500.

36. Scholey, A. et al., 'Chewing Gum Alleviates Negative Mood and Reduces Cortisol during Acute Laboratory Psychological Stress', *Physiology & Behavior* 97, no. 3–4 (June 2009): pp.304–12.

## Chapter 4

1. Unlu, N. Z. et al., 'Carotenoid Absorption from Salad and Salsa by Humans is Enhanced by the Addition of Avocado or Avocado Oil', *Journal of Nutrition* 135, no. 3 (March 2005): pp.431–6.

2. Johnston, C. S. et al., 'Vinegar: Medicinal Uses and Antiglycemic Effect', *Mescape General Medicine* 8, no. 2 (30 May 2006): p.61.

3. Tedong, L. et al., 'Hydro-Ethanolic Extract of Cashew Tree (Anacardium Occidentale) Nut and Its Principal Compound, Anacardic Acid, Stimulate Glucose Uptake in C2C12 Muscle Cells', *Molecular Nutrition and Food Research* 54, no. 12 (December 2010): pp.1753–62.

4. Kamil, A. et al., 'Health Benefits of Almonds Beyond Cholesterol Reduction', *Journal of Agricultural and Food Chemistry* (17 February 2012).

5.  Russo, M. et al., 'The Flavonoid Quercetin in Disease Prevention and Therapy', *Biochemical Pharmacology* 83, no. 1 (1 January 2012): pp.6–15.

6.  Mellen, P. B. et al., 'Whole Grain Intake and Cardiovascular Disease: A Meta-Analysis', *Nutrition, Metabolism and Cardiovascular Diseases* 18, no. 4 (May 2008): pp.283–90.

7.  Reis, C. E. et al., 'Ground Roasted Peanuts Leads to a Lower Post-Prandial Glycemic Response Than Raw Peanuts', *Nutrition Hospital* 26, no. 4 (July–August, 2011): pp.745–51.

8.  Oude Griep, L. M. et al., 'Colors of Fruit and Vegetables and 10-Year Incidence of Stroke', *Stroke* 42, no. 11 (November 2011): pp.3190–95.

9.  Shardell, M. D. et al., 'Low-Serum Carotenoid Concentrations and Carotenoid Interactions Predict Mortality in US Adults: The Third National Health and Nutrition Examination Survey', *Nutrition Research* 31, no. 3 (March 2011): pp.178–89.

10. Butt, M. S. et al., 'Black Pepper and Health Claims: A Comprehensive Treatise', *Critical Reviews in Food Science and Nutrition* 53, no. 9 (2013): pp.875–86.

11. Russell, F. D. et al., 'Distinguishing Health Benefits of Eicosapentaenoic and Docosahexaenoic Acids', *Marine Drugs* 10, no. 11 (13 November 2012): pp.2535–59.

12. Ludy, M. J. et al., 'The Effects of Capsaicin and Capsiate on Energy Balance: Critical Review and Meta-Analyses of Studies in Humans', *Chemical Senses* 37, no. 2 (February 2012): pp.103–21.

13. Ratliff, J. et al., 'Consuming Eggs for Breakfast Influences Plasma Glucose and Ghrelin, While Reducing Energy Intake During the Next 24 Hours in Adult Men', *Nutrition Research* 30, no. 2 (February 2010): pp.96–103.

14. Xu, Y. et al., 'Effect of Dietary Supplementation with White Button Mushrooms on Host Resistance to Influenza Infection and Immune Function in Mice', *British Journal of Nutrition* 109, no. 6 (28 March 2013): pp.1052–61.

15. Zhao, S. et al. 'Intakes of Apples or Apple Polyphenols Decrease Plasma Values for Oxidized Low-Density Lipoprotein/Beta 2-Glycoprotein I Complex.' *Journal of Funtional Foods* (January 2013): pp.493–497.

16. Hettiaratchi, U. P. et al., 'Chemical Compositions and Glycemic Responses to Banana Varieties', *International Journal of Food Sciences and Nutrition* 62, no. 4 (June 2011): pp.307–9.

17. Katz, D. L. et al., 'Cocoa and Chocolate in Human Health and Disease', *Antioxidants and Redox Signaling* 15, no. 10 (November 2011): pp.2779–811.

18. Patel, B. P. et al., 'An After-School Snack of Raisins Lowers Cumulative Food Intake in Young Children', *Journal of Food Science* 78, no. S1 (June 2013): pp.A5–A10.

19. Cesar, T. B. et al., 'Orange Juice Decreases Low-Density Lipoprotein Cholesterol in Hypercholesterolemic Subjects and Improves Lipid Transfer to High-Density Lipoprotein in Normal and Hypercholesterolemic Subjects', *Nutrition Research* 30, no. 10 (October 2010): pp.689–94.

20. Kurowska, E. M. et al., 'HDL-Cholesterol-Raising Effect of Orange Juice in Subjects with Hypercholesterolemia', *American Journal of Clinical Nutrition* 72, no. 5 (November 2000): pp.1095–100.

21. Zhang, Y. et al., 'Cherry Consumption and Decreased Risk of Recurrent Gout Attacks', *Arthritis and Rheumatism* 64, no. 12 (December 2012): pp.4004–11.

22. Kelley, D. S. et al., 'Sweet Bing Cherries Lower Circulating Concentrations of Markers for Chronic Inflammatory Diseases in Healthy Humans', *Journal of Nutrition* 143, no. 3 (March 2013): pp.340–44.

23. Howatson, G. et al., 'Effect of Tart Cherry Juice (Prunus Cerasus) on Melatonin Levels and Enhanced Sleep Quality', *European Journal of Nutrition* 51, no. 8 (December 2012): pp.909–16.

24. Moazzami, A. A. et al., 'Metabolomics Reveals the Metabolic Shifts Following an Intervention with Rye Bread in Postmenopausal Women – A Randomized Control Trial', *Nutrition Journal* 11 (October 2012): p.88.

25. Basu, A. et al., 'Strawberries Decrease Atherosclerotic Markers in Subjects with Metabolic Syndrome.' *Nutrition Research* 30, no. 7 (July 2010): pp.462–9.

26. Nguyen, V. et al., 'Popcorn Is More Satiating Than Potato Chips in Normal-Weight Adults', *Nutrition Journal* 11 (14 September 2012): p.71.

## Chapter 5

1. Bhutani, S. et al., 'Alternate Day Fasting and Endurance Exercise Combine to Reduce Body Weight and Favorably Alter Plasma Lipids on Obese Humans', *Obesity* (14 February 2013).
2. Bassett, D. R. Jr. et al., 'Pedometer-Measured Physical Activity and Health Behaviors in U.S. Adults', *Medicine and Science in Sports and Exercise* 42, no. 10 (October 2010): pp.1819–25.
3. Hultquist, C. N. et al., 'Comparison of Walking Recommendations in Previously Inactive Women', *Medicine and Science in Sports and Exercise* 37, no. 4 (April 2005): pp.676–83.
4. Tudor-Locke, C. et al., 'The Relationship between Pedometer-Determined Ambulatory Activity and Body Composition Variables', *International Journal of Obesity and Related Metabolic Disorders* 25, no. 11 (November 2001):pp.1571–8.
5. Bravata, D. M. 'Using Pedometers to Increase Physical Activity and Improve Health: A Systematic Review', *Journal of the American Medical Association* 298, no. 19 (21 November 2007): pp.2296–304.
6. Croteau, K. A., 'Strategies Used to Increase Lifestyle Physical Activity in a Pedometer-Based Intervention', *Journal of Allied Health* 33, no. 4 (Winter 2004): pp.278–81.
7. Steeves, J. A. et al., 'Can Sedentary Behavior Be Made More Active? A Randomized Pilot Study of TV Commercial Stepping Versus Walking', *International Journal of Behavioral Nutrition and Physical Activity* 9 (6 August 2012): p.95.

## Chapter 6

1. 'Obesity Week 2013', a presentation at the yearly scientific conference of the American Society for Metabolic and Bariatric Surgery, which publishes the journal *Obesity*, of first-year results from a three-year study sponsored by the National Institutes of Health.
2. Mekary, R. A. et al., 'Physical Activity in Relation to Long-Term Weight Maintenance After Intentional Weight Loss in Premenopausal Women', *Obesity* 18, no. 1 (January 2010): pp.167–74.

3. Robinson, E. et al., 'Eating Attentively: A Systematic Review and Meta-Analysis of the Effect of Food Intake Memory and Awareness on Eating', *American Journal of Clinical Nutrition* 97, no. 4 (April 2013): pp.728–42.

4. Beshara, M. et al., 'Does Mindfulness Matter? Everyday Mindfulness, Mindful Eating and Self-Reported Serving Size of Energy Dense Foods Among a Sample of South Australian Adults', *Appetite* 67 (August 2013): pp.25–9.

5. Alberts, H. J. et al., 'Dealing with Problematic Eating Behaviour: The Effects of a Mindfulness-Based Intervention on Eating Behaviour, Food Cravings, Dichotomous Thinking and Body Image Concern', *Appetite* 58, no. 3 (June 2012): pp.847–51.

6. Paolini, B. et al., 'Coping with Brief Periods of Food Restriction: Mindfulness Matters', *Frontiers in Aging Neuroscience* 4 (2012): p.13.

7. Daubenmier, J. et al., 'Mindfulness Intervention for Stress Eating to Reduce Cortisol and Abdominal Fat Among Overweight and Obese Women: An Exploratory Randomized Controlled Study', *Journal of Obesity* (2011): Article ID 651936.

8. Duffey, K. J. et al., 'Energy Density, Portion Size, and Eating Occasions: Contributions to Increased Energy Intake in the United States, 1977–2006', *PLoS Medicine* 8, no. 6 (June 2011): e1001050.

9. Wansink, B., et al., 'Portion Size Me: Downsizing Our Consumption Norms', *Journal of the American Dietetic Association* 107, no. 7 (July 2007): pp.1103–6.

10. Kesman, R. L. et al., 'Portion Control for the Treatment of Obesity in the Primary Care Setting', *BMC Research Notes* 4 (9 September 2011): p.346.

11. Pedersen, S. D. et al., 'Portion Control Plate for Weight Loss in Obese Patients with Type 2 Diabetes Mellitus: A Controlled Clinical Trial', *Archives of Internal Medicine* 167, no. 12 (June 2007): pp.1277–83.

12. Rolls, B. J. et al., 'Portion Size Can Be Used Strategically to Increase Vegetable Consumption in Adults', *American Journal of Clinical Nutrition* 91, no. 4 (April 2010): pp.913–22.

13. Van Kleef, E. et al., 'Serving Bowl Selection Biases the Amount of Food Served', *Journal of Nutrition Education and Behavior* 44, no. 1 (January–February 2012): pp.66–70.

14. Stroebele, N. et al., 'Do Calorie-Controlled Portion Sizes of Snacks Reduce Energy Intake?' *Appetite* 52, no. 3 (June 2009): pp.793–6.

15. Diliberti, N. et al., 'Increased Portion Size Leads to Increased Energy Intake in a Restaurant Meal', *Obesity* 12, no. 3 (March 2004): pp.562–568.

16. Condrasky, M. et al., 'Chefs' Opinions of Restaurant Portion Sizes', *Obesity* 15, no. 8 (August 2007): pp.2086–94.

17. Rolls, B. J. et al., 'Portion Size Can Be Used Strategically to Increase Vegetable Consumption in Adults', *American Journal of Clinical Nutrition* 91, no. 4 (April 2010): pp.913–22.

18. Hogenkamp, P. S. et al., 'Acute Sleep Deprivation Increases Portion Size and Affects Food Choice in Young Men', *Psychoneuroendocrinology* 38, no, 9 (September 2013): pp.1668–74.

# Index

A

adaptive thermogenesis 162
afternoon snacks 61
alcohol consumption 68–70
allergies 102
almonds
    almond-cherry smoothie 133
    Asian chicken salad 104–5
    health benefits of 100–1
    mango chicken salad 100
    scallops with pineapple salsa
        119–20
alpha-carotene 112
alternate-day fasting 17, 19, 85
alternate-day modified fasting
    (ADMF) 19, 26
Alzheimer's 114
American Association of Drugless
    Practitioners 2
*American Journal of Clinical
    Nutrition* 23–5, 57, 132, 176, 182,
    184
*American Journal of Physiology:
    Regulatory, Integrative and
    Comparative Physiology* 61
*American Journal of Preventative
    Medicine* 44
American Medical Association
    (AMA) 8
animals, diet research on 16–17
*Annals of Behavioral Medicine* 47
antioxidants 102, 129
anxiety 177

*Appetite* (journal) 66, 70, 74, 176
appetite
    gum chewing to reduce 74
    increased by diet soda 66–7
    water consumption and 64
    *see also* hunger
apples
    apple dippers 130
    BBQ pork chops with apple-
        topped sweet potato 112
    ham, apple and cheddar
        sandwich 98
    health benefits of 108, 125
    pork chop with sautéed apples
        and onions 124–5
apps, calorie-counting 173
*Archives of Internal Medicine* 181
artificial sweeteners 66, 67–8
Asian chicken salad 104–5
aspartame 68
Atkins Diet 14, 54
attentive eating *see* mindful eating
avocados
    chicken and bean quesadillas
        124
    health benefits of 124
    kidney bean and corn salad 97
    turkey and avocado sandwich 96

B

bacon 121
    BBQ bacon and pineapple pizza
        123

chicken and bacon lettuce wraps
  106
egg and cheese casserole 121
bagels
  berry bagel 131
  cinnamon bagel with orange
    spread 132
  turkey and cranberry bagel 102
bananas
  banana with crunchy berry
    topping 135–6
  and blood sugar 128
  PB&B square 128
basil: tomato-basil melt 132
Baumeister, Roy 148
BBQ bacon and pineapple pizza 123
BBQ chicken and broccoli wrap 96
BBQ pork chops with apple-topped
  sweet potato 112
BBQ salmon with mango salsa 115
beans
  chicken and bean quesadillas 124
  chicken enchiladas 111
  chicken nachos 118
  corn and bean burrito 106–7
  edamame pasta salad 104
  ham and butter bean soup 103
  health benefits of 108
  kidney bean and corn salad 97
  preparing 127
  sautéed prawns with kale and
    pine nuts 118
  spicy beef chilli 107–8
  spicy sausage and rice 126–7
  tuna and white bean salad 101
beef 174
  cheesy burger 113–14
  mini meat loaf with mashed
    potatoes 117
  roast beef roll 98
  roast beef with cucumber sauce
    108
  sirloin steak with mushroom
    sauce 121–2
  spaghetti and meatballs 110
  spicy beef chilli 107–8
  steak and peppers 112–13
  steak tacos 125
beer 69
belly fat 142, 167–8

berries 128
  banana with crunchy berry
    topping 135–6
  berries with fruit dip 136
  berry bagel 131
  frozen berry lolly 127
binge eating 144
  preventing 84–5
blood pressure 20, 25, 30–1, 102,
  114, 128, 129
blueberries 128
  frozen berry lolly 127
body mass index (BMI)
  calculating 22–3
  EOD Diet and 24
  exercise and 146–7
  main categories of 22
  overweight and obese 8, 22
  self-weighing and 46
boredom, eating and 177
bowls, size of 182–3
brand-name products 92
bread
  garden fresh toast 130
  ham, apple and cheddar
    sandwich 98
  open-faced cucumber sandwich
    133
  pepperoni French bread pizza
    110–11
  roast beef roll 98
  strawberries and cream toast 133
  turkey and avocado sandwich
    96
breakfast, skipping on Diet Day 49
*British Journal of Nutrition* 122
broccoli 134
  BBQ chicken and broccoli wrap
    96
  loaded baked potato 107
bromelain 105
Brussels sprouts 134
budgets, food 180
burgers, cheesy 113–14
burrito, corn and bean 106–7
butter beans: ham and butter bean
  soup 103
buttermilk: herby crumble-crusted
  cod 109–10

C
C-reactive protein 134
cabbage 134
caffeine 70–2
calcium 99, 133
calories
    counting 49–51, 172–4
    dietary struggle with 39–40
    EOD Diet 4–5, 18, 42–3
    EOD Success Programme 164–5,
        166–7
    hunger and need for 4
    intake on Feast Days 82, 83
    modified fasts and 18
    per pound of food 173–4
    RDA for men and women 41
    ready meals 93
    research on restricting 16–17
    restaurant meals and 59–60
    scientific explanation of 39
    scientific research on restriction
        of 16–17
    self-weighing and intake of 45
    traditional diets and calorie
        restriction 41
    water consumption and 64–5
cancer 110, 119, 134
    and calorie restriction 16
    EOD Diet and 32
cannellini beans
    chicken enchiladas 111
    sautéed prawns with kale and
        pine nuts 118
    tuna and white bean salad 101
carbohydrates, refined 174
cardiovascular disease *see* heart
    disease
carrots
    carrot sticks 129
    crackers with soft cheese and
        grated carrot 135
cashews
    chicken and cashew coleslaw 99
    health benefits of 99
casserole, egg and cheese 121
catechins 70–1
celery: mango chicken salad 100
cereal
    banana with crunchy berry
        topping 135–6

chocolate yogurt sundae 131
    sweet and salty snack mix 136
    trail mix 129
cheese 92, 121
    BBQ bacon and pineapple pizza
        123
    cheesy burger 113–14
    chicken and bean quesadillas 124
    chicken enchiladas 111
    chicken nachos 118
    chicken Parmesan 114
    corn and bean burrito 106–7
    egg and cheese casserole 121
    fruit with cheese spread 128
    ham, apple and cheddar
        sandwich 98
    ham and cheese spirals 134
    Mediterranean tuna-topped
        tomato 109
    pepperoni French bread pizza
        110–11
    roast beef roll 98
    steak tacos 125
    strawberries and cream toast 133
    taco salad 99
    tomato-basil melt 132
    tomatoes, peppers and cheese
        130
    tuna and white bean salad 101
    turkey and cranberry bagel 102
    *see also* cottage cheese; soft
        cheese
cherries
    almond-cherry smoothie 133
    health benefits of 133–4
chewing gum 72–5, 171
chicken 174
    Asian chicken salad 104–5
    BBQ chicken and broccoli wrap
        96
    chicken and bacon lettuce wraps
        106
    chicken and bean quesadillas 124
    chicken and cashew coleslaw 99
    chicken and pasta soup 103
    chicken cacciatore 122–3
    chicken enchiladas 111
    chicken nachos 118
    chicken Parmesan 114
    chicken stir-fry 115–16

chicken with roasted Dijon
potatoes 125–6
chicken with spinach and
tomatoes 119
mango chicken salad 100
taco salad 99
Thai noodle salad 105–6
chickpeas: Italian quinoa salad 95
children and the EOD Diet 32
chilli, spicy beef 107–8
chocolate
chocolate stack 129
chocolate yogurt sundae 131
dark chocolate 129
cholesterol 20, 24–5, 30, 31, 84, 108,
110
HDL 142
LDL 102, 125, 129, 132, 136, 142,
168
cinnamon
cinnamon bagel with orange
spread 132
cinnamon tortilla strips 134–5
cod, herby crumble-crusted 109–10
coffee 70–2
coleslaw, chicken and cashew 99
cookbooks, low-calorie 172
cottage cheese
health benefits of 133
open-faced cucumber sandwich
133
courgettes
ham and butter bean soup 103
penne primavera 120
couscous 102
turkey couscous salad 101
crackers with soft cheese and grated
carrot 135
cranberries: turkey and cranberry
bagel 102
cravings 74, 176
cream sauce 116–17
crème fraîche: creamy dip with
peppers 135
crumpets: fruity crumpet sticks 131
cucumber
BBQ salmon with mango salsa
115
garden fresh toast 130
health benefits of 108

hummus cucumber boats 127
Italian quinoa salad 95
open-faced cucumber sandwich
133
roast beef with cucumber sauce
108
tuna and white bean salad 101
*Current Medical Research and
Opinion* 74–5

D
dairy products
USDA recommendation for 182
*see also* cheese; milk
Davis, Allison P. 85–7
Davy, Brenda 64
depression 177
deprivation, dietary 3–4
DHA (docosahexaenoic acid) 56
diabetes 42, 110
diet soda and 67
EOD Diet and 32
snacks 128
*Diabetes Care* 67, 68
Diet Day 39–78
100-calorie snacks 127–36
400-calorie dinners 109–27
400-calorie lunches 95–109
alcohol consumption on 68–70
brand-based products 92
caloric intake on 41, 42–3, 49–50
characteristics of 90–2
cheating on 77–8
and chewing gum 72–5
coffee consumption 70–2
drinking water before meals 64
easing hunger 63–75
eating lunch or dinner 48–9
eating meals out 59–60
fat content of foods on 32–4,
55–6
hunger experienced on 28, 41–2
mini-meals 51–2
planning your meals 51
published study about 27–9
ready meals 50–1, 93
recipes for 50, 89–136
simplicity of 78
snacks 60–1, 127–36
tea consumption 70–2

tips for succeeding on 44–61
water consumption 64–5
weighing yourself 44–7
when to exercise 75, 143–4
*see also* Feast Day; Success Days
diets
Atkins Diet 14, 54
eating restrictions on 54
failure of traditional 1–2, 3–4, 163
Mediterranean diet 56, 120
Ornish Diet 14, 54
Paleo Diet 54
scientific studies on popular 14
dinner
400-calorie dinners 109–27
BBQ bacon and pineapple pizza
123
BBQ pork chops with apple-
topped sweet potato 112
BBQ salmon with mango salsa
115
cheesy burger 113–14
chicken and bean quesadillas 124
chicken cacciatore 122–3
chicken nachos 118
chicken Parmesan 114
chicken with roasted Dijon
potatoes 125–6
chicken with spinach and
tomatoes 119
eating on Diet Day 48–9
egg and cheese casserole 121
herby crumble-crusted cod
109–10
mini meat loaf with mashed
potatoes 117
pasta with cream sauce 116–17
penne primavera 120
pork chop with sautéed apples
and onions 124–5
ravioli with vegetables 116
rigatoni in tomato cream sauce
123
sautéed prawns with kale and
pine nuts 118
scallops with pineapple salsa
119–20
sirloin steak with mushroom
sauce 121–2
spaghetti and meatballs 110
spicy sausage and rice 126–7
steak and peppers 112–13
steak tacos 125
stir-fry chicken 115–16
*see also* lunch
dips
berries with fruit dip 136
creamy dip with peppers 135
diseases
artificial sweeteners and 67
obesity recognized as 8
*see also* cancer; diabetes; heart
disease, *etc*
distracted eating 174–6
docosahexaenoic acid (DHA) 56
drinks
almond-cherry smoothie 133
fizzy 66–7
*see also* water consumption

E
*Eat, Fast, and Live Longer* (BBC) 26
eating
changing your pattern of 87
eating out 59–60, 91
emotional eating 144, 174–6
mindful eating 174–9
portion control for 179–84
edamame pasta salad 104
eggs 121
egg and cheese casserole 121
Eichele, Gerd 57–8
eicosapentaenoic acid (EPA) 56
*Elle* 85
emotional eating 144, 174–6
emotional hunger cues 85
enchiladas, chicken 111
EPA (eicosapentaenoic acid) 56
European Food Safety Authority
(EFSA) 68
Every-Other-Day (EOD) Diet
basic rule of 4, 40
caloric intake on 5, 18, 20, 42–3
cheating on 24, 34, 77–8
exercise with 34–5, 139–42
heart disease and 29–31
recipes for 89–136
research published on 23–37
safety of 31–2
satisfaction rating 28

scientific studies on 14–15, 18–37
snacks for 60–1
traditional diets vs. EOD 2
weight loss on 23–4, 37–8
*see also* Diet Day; Feast Day;
    Success Day
Every-Other-Day (EOD) Success
    Programme 38, 163–87
    caloric intake 164–5, 166–7, 172–4
    continuing good habits 170–1
    mindful eating 174–9
    portion control 179–84
    results of studies on 36, 166–7
    Success Days 164–5
exercise 137–59
    benefits of regular 137–9
    best times for on Diet Day 75,
        143–4, 149
    EOD Diet combined with 34–5,
        139–42
    EOD Success Programme and
        170–1
    five secrets of regular 147–50
    increasing your daily 152–7
    pedometer-based programme
        150–9
    planning 148–9
    recommended levels of 145
    self-efficacy related to 158
    walking 145–7, 150–9
    weight loss and 140–1
external eating 174–6

F
fast day *see* Diet Day
fast-food restaurants 59–60, 180
fasting
    alternate-day 17, 19
    modified alternate-day 2, 19
fat, tummy 33, 36, 142, 167–8
fat loss *see* weight loss
fatigue, during exercise 102
fats 121, 174
    benefits of consuming 56–7
    consumption on Diet Day 33–4,
        55–6
    consumption on Feast Day 87
    cooking without 113
    high-fat foods 33–4, 55–6, 87
    low-fat diet 33

monounsaturated 124
omega-3 56, 115
saturated 56–7
traditional diets and 54
Feast Day 79–88
    basic rule of 79
    caloric intake on 5, 82, 83
    comments from dieters about
        80–2
    enjoying yourself on 87–8
    EOD Success Programme 165
    food consumption on 83–4, 87–8
    high-fat foods eaten on 87
    surprising science of 82–5
    *see also* Diet Day; Success Day
feta cheese
    edamame pasta salad 104
    Mediterranean tuna-topped
        tomato 109
    tuna and white bean salad 101
fish
    BBQ salmon with mango salsa
        115
    health benefits of 56, 115
    herby crumble-crusted cod
        109–10
    Italian quinoa salad 95
    Mediterranean tuna-topped
        tomato 109
    tuna and white bean salad 101
    tuna salad snack 131
Fitbit pedometer 151
fizzy drinks 66–7
free radicals 132
French bread: pepperoni French
    bread pizza 110–11
fruit
    berries with fruit dip 136
    calories per pound in 173
    frozen berry lolly 127
    fruit with cheese spread 128
    fruity crumpet sticks 131
    health benefits of 108
    increasing portions of 182
    *see also* apples; bananas, *etc*
fullness, feeling of 179

G
garden fresh toast 130
garlic, health benefits of 119

gherkins: turkey-lettuce rolls 136
gherlin 163
glucagon-like peptide 1 (GLP-1) 67
goal setting 157
Gottlieb, Bill 2, 46
   *Breakthroughs in Natural*
      *Healing* 72
   *The Natural Fat-Loss Pharmacy*
      70
gout 133
Gower, Paul 53–4
green tea 70–2
gum chewing 72–5, 171

**H**
'Halftime Diet' (*Elle*) 85
ham
   ham, apple and cheddar
      sandwich 98
   ham and butter bean soup 103
   ham and cheese spirals 134
   ham and pear wrap 102
   ham and rice salad 105
   loaded baked potato 107
   *see also* pork recipes
haricot beans
   sautéed prawns with kale and
      pine nuts 118
   tuna and white bean salad 101
Harvard School of Public Health 56,
   70
HDL cholesterol 142
heart attacks 120
heart disease 134
   EOD Diet and 29–31, 32, 37
   EOD Success Programme and
      168
   exercise and 142
   fighting and preventing 42, 110,
      114, 119, 129
   saturated fat and 56–7
   and wholegrains 105
heart rate 25
Hellerstein, Marc 16
herbs
   health benefits of 110
   herby crumble-crusted cod
      109–10
Hill, James 146, 154–6
hummus

   calories in 100
   garden fresh toast 130
   hummus cucumber boats 127
   turkey and hummus wrap 100
hunger
   coffee or tea for controlling 70
   experienced on Diet Day 28, 41–2
   gum chewing to reduce 72–5
   hormones controlling 163
   and popcorn 136
   protein for reducing 52–3
   recognizing physical signs of 178
   strategies for easing 63–75
   traditional diets and 4
   tuning in to real 85
   water consumption and 64, 171
Hussein, Paul 25–7

**I**
infusion pitchers 65–6
*International Journal of Behavioral*
   *Medicine* 45
*International Journal of Food*
   *Sciences and Nutrition* 128
*International Journal of Obesity* 35,
   71
Italian quinoa salad 95

**J**
jalapeño peppers 118
jam: berries with fruit dip 136
*Journal of the Academy of Nutrition*
   *and Dietetics* 63
*Journal of the American Dietetic*
   *Association* 61, 63
*Journal of the American Medical*
   *Association* 14
*Journal of Clinical Endocrinology*
   *and Metabolism* 64–5
*Journal of Nutrition* 71
*Journal of Nutrition Education and*
   *Behavior* 182
jumbo-sized portions 180
junk food 174

**K**
kale 134
   health benefits of 104
   sautéed prawns with kale and
      pine nuts 118

turkey and orzo soup 103–4
Karpinske, Stephanie 90
kidney beans
    chicken enchiladas 111
    health benefits of 108
    kidney bean and corn salad 97
    spicy beef chilli 107–8
    spicy sausage and rice 126–7
kidney disease 67
Klempel, Dr Monica 86

L
Lang, Fred 47–8
LDL (low-density lipoprotein)
    cholesterol *see* cholesterol
lean body mass 18, 31–2
leptin 163
lettuce 99
    chicken and bacon lettuce wraps
        106
    corn and bean burrito 106–7
    ham and cheese spirals 134
    ham and rice salad 105
    steak tacos 125
    turkey and cranberry bagel 102
    turkey-lettuce rolls 136
leukaemia 67
lifestyle, changes to 156–7
lipidophobia 55
loaded baked potato 107
lollies, frozen berry 127
low-density lipoprotein (LDL)
    cholesterol *see* cholesterol
lunch
    400-calorie 95–109
    Asian chicken salad 104–5
    BBQ chicken and broccoli wrap
        96
    chicken and bacon lettuce wraps
        106
    chicken and cashew coleslaw 99
    chicken and pasta soup 103
    corn and bean burrito 106–7
    eating on Diet Day 48–9
    edamame pasta salad 104
    ham, apple and cheddar
        sandwich 98
    ham and butter bean soup 103
    ham and pear wrap 102
    ham and rice salad 105

Italian quinoa salad 95
kidney bean and corn salad 97
loaded baked potato 107
mango chicken salad 100
Mediterranean tuna-topped
    tomato 109
roast beef roll 98
roast beef with cucumber sauce
    108
spicy beef chilli 107–8
taco salad 99
Thai noodle salad 105–6
tortellini salad 97
tuna and white bean salad 101
turkey and avocado sandwich 96
turkey and cranberry bagel 102
turkey and hummus wrap 100
turkey and orzo soup 103–4
turkey couscous salad 101
    *see also* dinner
lycopene 96

M
McDonald's 60
mangetout
    chicken and cashew coleslaw 99
    tortellini salad 97
mangoes
    BBQ salmon with mango salsa
        115
    mango chicken salad 100
marinades 126
Marshfield Clinic Research
    Foundation 45
Martin Ginis, Kathleen 147–8
May, Michelle, *Eat What You Love,
    Love What You Eat* 177–9
mayonnaise 92
meals, planning Diet Day 51
meat loaf with mashed potatoes 117
meatballs, spaghetti and 110
medication, EOD Diet and 32
Mediterranean diet 56, 120
Mediterranean tuna-topped tomato
    109
Melanson, Kathleen 72, 73
men, and calorie requirement 41
*Metabolism* (journal) 32–4
metabolism
    effect of weight loss on 162–3

resetting with EOD Diet 84
  water consumption and 65
mid-morning snacks 61
milk 72
mindful eating 174–9
  guidelines for 177–9
  research supporting 176–7
Minneapolis Heart Institute 44–5
modified alternate-day fasting 2, 19
monounsaturated fat 124
mood, and exercise 149
Mosley, Michael 26
mozzarella cheese
  chicken Parmesan 114
  ham and cheese spirals 134
  pepperoni French bread pizza
    110–11
  tomato-basil melt 132
  tomatoes, peppers and cheese
    130
muffins: tomato-basil melt 132
muscle mass
  EOD Diet and 24, 42, 141–2, 167
  increasing with exercise 141–2
  losing while dieting 18, 163, 167
mushrooms
  chicken cacciatore 122–3
  health benefits of 122
  penne primavera 120
  pepperoni French bread pizza
    110–11
  sirloin steak with mushroom
    sauce 121–2
  turkey and orzo soup 103–4
mustard, health benefits 134

N
nachos, chicken 118
National Institutes of Health (NIH)
  14, 37, 83, 166, 168
National Weight Control Registry
  146
*New England Journal of Medicine*
  56, 120
NHS Choices, BMI calculator 22–3
nighttime snacks 61
nitric oxide 104
noodles: Thai noodle salad 105–6
Novick, Jeffrey 173
*Nutrition Journal* 27–9, 139

nuts 174
  almond-cherry smoothie 133
  Asian chicken salad 104–5
  chicken and cashew coleslaw 99
  health benefits of 56, 99, 100–1
  mango chicken salad 100
  PB&B square 128
  sautéed prawns with kale and
    pine nuts 118
  scallops with pineapple salsa
    119–20
  Thai noodle salad 105–6

O
Oakland Research Institute 57
obesity
  BMI indicating 8, 22
  diet soda and risk of 67
  and green tea catechins 71
  health problems linked to 8–9
  lack of exercise related to 146–7
  medical designation of 8
  worldwide prevalence of 9
*Obesity* (journal) 29–31, 34–5, 46,
  52, 67, 70, 142, 183
*Obesity Research* 71, 183
Obesity Society, 'ObesityWeek'
  (2013) 35–7, 166
oils 174
  olive oil 56, 120
olives
  chicken with spinach and
    tomatoes 119
  Mediterranean tuna-topped
    tomato 109
  roast beef roll 98
omega-3 fatty acids 56, 115
Omron pedometers 151
onions
  mango chicken salad 100
  pork chop with sauteed apples
    and onions 124–5
  red onions 102
oranges
  cinnamon bagel with orange
    spread 132
  health benefits of 132
  turkey couscous salad 101
oregano, health benefits of 110
orientin 132

Ornish Diet 14, 54
orzo: turkey and orzo soup 103–4
overeating 143
    on EOD 27–8
overweight
    BMI indicating 8, 22
    medical designation of 8
    percentage of population as 9
    *see also* obesity

P
package/beverage size 183
Paleo Diet 54
parfait, Greek yogurt 128–9
Parmesan, chicken 114
parsley, health benefits of 110
pasta
    chicken and pasta soup 103
    chicken cacciatore 122–3
    edamame pasta salad 104
    fresh 117
    pasta with cream sauce 116–17
    penne primavera 120
    ravioli with vegetables 116
    rigatoni in tomato cream sauce
        123
    spaghetti and meatballs 110
    tortellini salad 97
    tuna and white bean salad 101
    turkey and orzo soup 103–4
    types of 120
PB&B square 128
peanut butter
    chocolate stack 129
    PB&B square 128
peanuts
    health benefits of 106
    Thai noodle salad 105–6
pears
    ham and pear wrap 102
    health benefits of 108
peas
    ham and rice salad 105
    pasta with cream sauce 116–17
pedometer-based walking
    programme 150–9
    buying a pedometer 151–2
    daily steps calculation 152–4
    increasing your steps 153–5
    making small changes 156–7

    self-efficacy related to 158
    *see also* walking
pepper, black 114
pepperoni French bread pizza
    110–11
peppers
    Asian chicken salad 104–5
    chicken cacciatore 122–3
    chicken nachos 118
    creamy dip with peppers 135
    edamame pasta salad 104
    garden fresh toast 130
    ham and butter bean soup 103
    kidney bean and corn salad 97
    penne primavera 120
    roast beef roll 98
    steak and peppers 112–13
    taco salad 99
    Thai noodle salad 105–6
    tomatoes, peppers and cheese
        130
    tortellini salad 97
physical activity
    Diet Day vs. Feast Day 28–9
    weight loss related to 146–7,
        170–1
    *see also* exercise
phytoestrogens 104
pine nuts, sautéed prawns with kale
    and 118
pineapple
    Asian chicken salad 104–5
    BBQ bacon and pineapple pizza
        123
    health benefits of 105
    scallops with pineapple salsa
        119–20
piperine 114
pitta breads: roast beef with
    cucumber sauce 108
pizza
    BBQ bacon and pineapple pizza
        123
    pepperoni French bread pizza
        110–11
planning
    Diet Day meals 51
    exercise 148–9
    planning meals 91
    plates for portion control 181–2

popcorn
and hunger 136
sweet and salty snack mix 136
pork
BBQ pork chops with apple-
topped sweet potato 112
pork chop with sauteed apples
and onions 124–5
*see also* ham recipes
portion control 176, 179–84
plates for 181–2
science-based tips for 181–4
potassium 107
potatoes
chicken with roasted Dijon
potatoes 125–6
health benefits of 107, 112
loaded baked potato 107
mini meat loaf with mashed
potatoes 117
poultry *see* chicken; turkey
prawns: sautéed prawns with kale
and pine nuts 118
pregnant women 32
protein 121, 174
lean vs. fatty 174
reducing hunger with 52–3

Q
quercetin 102
quesadillas, chicken and bean 124
quinoa salad, Italian 95

R
raisins
health benefits 129
trail mix cereal 129
ravioli with vegetables 116
Ravussin, Eric 18–19
ready meals 50–1, 93–5
refined carbohydrates 174
refried beans
chicken and bean quesadillas 124
corn and bean burrito 106–7
restaurants
Diet Day meals at 59–60
portion size 183–4
rice
Asian chicken salad 104–5
brown rice 105

chicken stir-fry 115–16
ham and rice salad 105
spicy sausage and rice 126–7
Richardson, Dr Caroline 151, 152–3,
157, 158
Rye Factor 135
Ryvita: mango chicken salad 100

S
SACN (Scientific Advisory
Committee on Nutrition) 41
salad dressings 92
salads
Asian chicken 104–5
chicken and cashew coleslaw 99
edamame pasta 104
ham and rice 105
Italian quinoa 95
kidney bean and corn 97
mango chicken 100
taco 99
Thai noodle 105–6
tortellini 97
tuna and white bean 101
tuna salad snack 131
turkey couscous salad 101
salmon
BBQ salmon with mango salsa
115
health benefits of 115
salsa
corn and bean burrito 106–7
creamy dip with peppers 135
mango 115
pineapple 119–20
spicy beef chilli 107–8
spicy sausage and rice 126–7
taco salad 99
salt 92, 103
sweet and salty snack mix 136
sandwiches
ham, apple and cheddar 98
open-faced cucumber 133
roast beef roll 98
turkey and avocado 96
*see also* bagels, wraps
saturated fat 56–7
sauces
cream 116–17
cucumber 108

mushroom 121–2
tomato cream 123
sausages: spicy sausage and rice
    126–7
scallops with pineapple salsa 119–20
Scientific Advisory Committee on
    Nutrition (SACN) 41
scientific studies 13–14
    on calorie restriction 16–17
    on EOD Diet 14–15, 18–37
    on popular diets 14
seafood 174
    sautéed prawns with kale and
        pine nuts 118
    scallops with pineapple salsa
        119–20
seeds 174
self-efficacy 158
senior citizens, and snacking 63
sleep and portion sizes 184
smoothie, almond-cherry 133
snacks
    100-calorie 127
    almond-cherry smoothie 133
    apple dippers 130
    benefits of 62–3
    berries with fruit dip 136
    berry bagel 131
    carrot sticks 129
    chocolate stack 129
    chocolate yogurt sundae 131
    cinnamon bagel with orange
        spread 132
    cinnamon tortilla strips 134–5
    creamy dip with peppers 135
    eating on Diet Day 60–1
    frozen berry lolly 127
    fruit with cheese spread 128
    fruity crumpet sticks 131
    garden fresh toast 130
    Greek yogurt parfait 128–9
    ham and cheese spirals 134
    hummus cucumber boats 127
    open-faced cucumber sandwich
        133
    PB&B square 128
    size considerations for 183
    strawberries and cream toast 133
    sweet and salty snack mix 136
    time of day for 61

tomato-basil melt 132
tomatoes, peppers and cheese
    130
trail mix cereal 129
tuna salad snack 131
turkey-lettuce rolls 136
soda, diet 66–7
soft cheese
    apple dippers 130
    cinnamon bagel with orange
        spread 132
    crackers with soft cheese and
        grated carrot 135
    fruity crumpet sticks 131
    ham and pear wrap 102
    pasta with cream sauce 116–17
soups
    chicken and pasta 103
    ham and butter bean 103
    turkey and orzo 103–4
soybeans: edamame pasta salad 104
spaghetti and meatballs 110
spicy beef chilli 107–8
spicy sausage and rice 126–7
spinach
    chicken with spinach and
        tomatoes 119
    ravioli with vegetables 116
    turkey and hummus wrap 100
starters, calories in 60
steak
    steak and peppers 112–13
    steak tacos 125
    steak with mushroom sauce
        121–2
step count
    calculating your daily 152–4
    increasing your daily 153–6
    *see also* walking
stevia 68
stir-fry, chicken 115–16
stock cubes 103
stomach shrinking 84
strawberries 128
    berries with fruit dip 136
    berry bagel 131
    chocolate stack 129
    frozen berry lolly 127
    Greek yogurt parfait 128–9
    health benefits of 136

strawberries and cream toast 133
stress
gum chewing to reduce 74–5
stress eating 175, 177
*Stroke: Journal of the American
Heart Association* 108
strokes 67, 108, 119, 120, 129
Success Days
caloric intake on 164–5, 166
drinking water 171
*see also* Every-Other-Day (EOD)
Success Programme
sucralose 68
sugar 72
sugar-free gum 72–5
sultanas: turkey couscous salad 101
sundae, chocolate yogurt 131
superfruits 128
sweet potatoes
BBQ pork chops with apple-
topped sweet potato 112
health benefits of 112
*see also* potatoes
sweetcorn
BBQ chicken and broccoli wrap
96
corn and bean burrito 106–7
kidney bean and corn salad 97
spicy sausage and rice 126–7
sweeteners, artificial 66, 67–8

T
tacos
steak tacos 125
taco salad 99
tea 70–2
teenagers and the EOD Diet 32
Thai noodle salad 105–6
toast
garden fresh toast 130
strawberries and cream toast 133
tomatoes
chicken and bacon lettuce wraps
106
chicken cacciatore 122–3
chicken enchiladas 111
chicken Parmesan 114
chicken with spinach and
tomatoes 119
edamame pasta salad 104

ham and rice salad 105
health benefits of 96
kidney bean and corn salad 97
Mediterranean tuna-topped
tomato 109
pepperoni French bread pizza
110–11
rigatoni in tomato cream sauce
123
spaghetti and meatballs 110
spicy beef chilli 107–8
steak tacos 125
tomato-basil melt 132
tomatoes, peppers and cheese
130
tuna salad snack 131
turkey and avocado sandwich 96
turkey and hummus wrap 100
tortellini salad 97
tortilla chips
chicken nachos 118
taco salad 99
tortillas: cinnamon tortilla strips
134–5
trail mix cereal 129
triglycerides 30, 31, 134
tummy fat 33, 36, 142, 167–8
tuna
calories in 101
Italian quinoa salad 95
Mediterranean tuna-topped
tomato 109
tuna and white bean salad 101
tuna salad snack 131
turkey
carrot sticks 129
spaghetti and meatballs 110
turkey and avocado sandwich 96
turkey and cranberry bagel 102
turkey and hummus wrap 100
turkey and orzo soup 103–4
turkey couscous salad 101
turkey-lettuce rolls 136
Twain, Mark 161

U
UK Chief Medical Officer, exercise
recommendations 145
UK Food Standards Agency 93

V
vegetables 94
    calories per pound in 173
    chicken and pasta soup 103
    chicken stir-fry 115–16
    health benefits of 108
    increasing portions of 182
    ravioli with vegetables 116
    *see also* carrots; potatoes, *etc*
very low-calorie diet (VLCD) 41
vicenin 132
vinegar 97
visceral fat 168
vitamin A 99
vitamin C 99
VLCD (very low-calorie diet) 41

W
walking 145–7
    increasing your daily 153–5
    pedometer-based programme
        150–9
    weight loss related to 146–7
    *see also* exercise
Wansink, Brian 183, 184
    *Mindless Eating: Why We Eat
        More Than We Think* 180–1
water consumption
    burning calories with 64–5
    easing hunger with 64, 171
    infusing water 65–6
    weight loss and 65
web resources, BMI calculator 22–3
weighing
    daily 44–7, 171
    self-weighing 44–7, 171
weight loss
    author's account of 5–8
    calorie restriction and 16–17
    coffee consumption and 70
    daily weighing and 44–5, 47
    EOD Diet and 23–4, 37–8

exercise and 140–1, 170–1
    gum chewing and 72–3
    high-fat diet and 55, 87
    maintaining 35–6, 167
    normal BMI 22
    regaining weight after 35–6,
        162–3
    snacks for maintaining 63
    tea consumption and 71
    water consumption and 65
weight maintenance
    calorie consumption for 41
    daily weighing and 45–6, 47
    EOD Success Programme and 36,
        166–9
    mindfulness and 177
    snacks and 63
    tea consumption and 71
Whigham, Leah 73–4
wholegrains 105, 136, 173
willpower 144, 148–50
wine 69
women, and calorie requirement 41
wraps
    BBQ chicken and broccoli 96
    ham and pear 102
    turkey and hummus 100
    *see also* sandwiches

Y
yogurt
    banana with crunchy berry
        topping 135–6
    berries with fruit dip 136
    chocolate yogurt sundae 131
    frozen berry lolly 127
    Greek yogurt parfait 128–9
    mango chicken salad 100

Z
Zone Diet 14, 54